no-fuss diabetes desserts

Fresh, Fast & Diabetes-Friendly Desserts

LINDA GASSENHEIMER

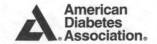

American Diabetes Association.

Director, Book Publishing, Abe Ogden; *Managing Editor,* Greg Guthrie; *Acquisitions Editor,* Victor Van Beuren; *Production Manager,* Melissa Sprott; *Composition,* ADA; *Production Services,* Cenveo Publisher Services, Inc.; *Cover Design,* Design Literate; *Printer,* United Graphics.

Printed in the United States of America
1 3 5 7 9 10 8 6 4 2

ADA titles may be purchased for business or promotional use or for special sales. To purchase more than 50 copies of this book at a discount, or for custom editions of this book with your logo, contact the American Diabetes Association at the address below, at booksales@diabetes.org, or by calling 703-299-2046.

American Diabetes Association
1701 North Beauregard Street
Alexandria, Virginia 22311

DOI: 10.2337/9781580405287

Library of Congress Cataloging-in-Publication Data
Gassenheimer, Linda.
 No-fuss diabetes desserts / by Linda Gassenheimer.
  pages cm
 Includes bibliographical references and index.
 ISBN 978-1-58040-528-7 (alk. paper) 1. Diabetes–Diet therapy–Recipes.
2. Desserts.
 I. American Diabetes Association. II. Title.
 RC662.G38 2014
 641.5'6314–dc23
                    2014000196

To my husband, Harold,
for his love,
constant enthusiasm for my work,
and support.

Contents

Acknowledgments

One of the best parts of writing a book is working with so many talented and friendly people. I'd like to thank them all for their enthusiastic support.

My biggest thank you goes to my husband, Harold, who encouraged me, helped me test every recipe, and spent hours helping me edit every word. His constant encouragement for all of my work has made this book a partnership.

Thank you to Abe Ogden, Director of Book Publishing at the American Diabetes Association, for his guidance and support. He worked closely with me to enable this book to come to life.

I'd also like to thank Greg Guthrie, Managing Editor at the American Diabetes Association, for his wonderful work in managing this book. Thanks also to Melissa Sprott, Production Manager, for creating the beautiful design for this book.

Thank you to Joseph Cooper and Bonnie Berman, hosts of *Topical Currents*, and to the staff at WLRN National Public Radio for their help and enthusiasm for my weekly "Food News and Views" segment.

I'd also like to thank my family, who have supported my projects and encouraged me every step of the way: my son James, his wife Patty, and their children Zachary, Jacob, and Haley; my son John, his wife Jill, and their children Jeffrey and Joanna; and my son Charles, his wife Lori, and their sons Daniel and Matthew; and my sister Roberta and her husband Robert.

And, finally, thank you to all of my readers and listeners who have written and called over the years. You have helped shape my ideas and made the solitary task of writing a two-way street.

Introduction:
No-Fuss Desserts

Looking for something sweet at the end of a meal? If you're like me, the meal isn't complete without dessert. It doesn't have to be elaborate, just something that's quick, easy, and delicious that won't break my calorie or carbohydrate bank. You'll find 60 desserts here with a variety of flavors and textures to fit your every mood. They take only minutes to prepare.

Thinking about a chocolate treat? Try the light-as-a-cloud Chocolate Mousse. Or maybe it's a rich chocolate you're craving– the Chocolate Pudding is creamy with a deep chocolate flavor. I love cookies and the Chocolate Chip Meringue Cookies are perfect for any occasion.

The mocha desserts blend coffee and chocolate together, creating a mouth-watering delight. The Mocha Fudge Cake takes only 8 minutes in the oven.

Take advantage of fruits when they're in season. They are ripened by the sun and full of flavor. Sweet strawberries, plump blueberries, fragrant mangoes, and ripe peaches are some of the fruits I have used here. Peach Crumble can be made partially in a microwave oven. Strawberry Frozen Yogurt Cup pairs fresh strawberries with frozen yogurt for a summer delight. Deep Dish Blueberry Cream has a sweet blueberry topping.

I used favorite flavor memories from my childhood to create the Banana Pudding and the Peanut Butter Apple "S'mores" recipes. They capture the essence of these old-time favorites, but with a new twist.

Shopping

The ingredients for these desserts can be found in a local supermarket. I've included a shopping list with what you need to buy and what staples to keep on hand. There's also a Shop Smart section added to the recipes to help you choose the best ingredients from the supermarket.

Enjoy these desserts with sweet dreams.

Shop Smart

To help assemble these desserts in minutes, I have designed these recipe using ingredients you can find at your supermarket. This guide isn't a specific recommendation of any particular brand. You can choose from the many options available. The key is to *shop smart* by looking at the nutrition information provided in this section. I have listed the items for which I have found a range of products with variations in calorie, fat, carbohydrate, or sodium content to guide you toward healthy options. You may not find these exact values. Use this information as a guideline for what you choose.

Many of these items can be kept on hand so that you only have to shop for a few fresh ingredients.

Look for the following:

- Dark chocolate chips with 70 calories, 3.0 g saturated fat, 9.0 g carbohydrates per 15 g

- Low-fat chocolate or strawberry frozen yogurt with 99 calories, 0.9 g saturated fat, 18.3 g carbohydrates per 1/2 cup

- Frozen, nonfat whipped topping (such as Cool Whip) with 7.5 calories, 1.5 g carbohydrates per tablespoon

- Grape jam with 56 calories, 13.8 g carbohydrates per tablespoon

- Sugar-free grape jam or orange marmalade with 18 calories, 7.5 g carbohydrates per tablespoon

- Low-fat yogurt with 154 calories, 3.8 g fat, 12.9 g protein, 17.3 g carbohydrates, 172 mg sodium per cup

- Low-fat Greek yogurt with 130 calories, 3.5 g fat, 7.0 g carbohydrates, 70 mg sodium per 6 ounces

- Nonfat yogurt with 97 calories, 0.3 g fat, 17.0 g carbohydrates, 133 mg sodium per cup

- Low-fat, no-salt-added cottage cheese with 163 calories, 2.3 g fat, 28.0 g protein, 6.1 g carbohydrates, 29 mg sodium per cup

- Nonfat ricotta cheese with 200 calories, 20.0 g protein, 20.0 g carbohydrates, 260 mg sodium per cup

- Pasteurized whole eggs for those desserts where the eggs are not cooked

- Pasteurized, liquid egg whites with 7.5 calories, 0 g fat, 1.6 g protein, 24 mg sodium per tablespoon

- Reduced-fat sour cream with 20 calories, 1.8 g fat, 0.4 g protein, 0.6 g carbohydrates, 13 mg sodium per tablespoon

- Vanilla soymilk with 131 calories, 4.3 g fat, 8.0 g protein, 15.3 g carbohydrates, 125 mg sodium per cup

- Sugar substitute of your choice (I have used several different brands in creating the recipes)

Fruit Fabulous

Cheddar Apples with Walnuts

*Cheese, apples, and walnuts make a perfect combination
for the end of your meal or any time.*

Helpful Hints

- Cut apple into wedges about 1/2-inch thick.
- Instead of Cheddar cheese cubes, you can shred the cheese over the apple slices.

> 1 apple, cut into wedges
> 1 tablespoon lemon juice
> 1/2 ounce reduced-fat Cheddar cheese, cubed
> 1 tablespoon unsalted walnuts halves

- Cut apples in half and remove the core. Cut each half into 3 wedges and toss in lemon juice. Arrange apples on a small dessert plate.

- Cut cheese into small cubes and place on the plate with the apple and walnuts.

Makes one serving.

*Exchanges/Choices: 1 fruit, 1 medium-fat protein
Per serving: Calories 141, Calories from Fat 54, Total Fat 6.0 g, Saturated Fat 1.1 g,
Monounsaturated Fat 1.0 g, Cholesterol 3 mg, Protein 4.9 g, Carbohydrates 19.6 g, Dietary
Fiber 3.5 g, Sugars 13.6 g, Sodium 125 mg, Potassium 191 mg, Phosphorus 109 mg*

Shopping List:

1 apple
1 lemon
1 small package reduced-fat Cheddar
   cheese
1 package unsalted walnut halves

Apple Fluff

Light and fresh tasting, this dessert is like biting into an apple-cinnamon cloud. It's especially good made with Granny Smith apples.

Helpful Hints

- Whole pasteurized eggs can be found in most supermarkets.
- Purée the apples in a food processor or force them through a sieve or strainer.
- To test if the egg whites form stiff peaks, lift beater with a little beaten egg white on it. The egg white should not move when shaken lightly.

1 cup apple chunks
1/2 cup water
1 tablespoon honey
Sugar substitute equivalent to 2 teaspoons sugar
1 teaspoon vanilla extract
1/2 teaspoon ground cinnamon
2 egg whites, separated from whole pasteurized eggs
1 tablespoon unsalted walnut pieces

- Peel and core the apples, cut into 1-inch pieces, and measure 1 cup. Add apples to a saucepan with the water, honey, and sugar substitute. Place over medium heat, bring to a simmer, lower heat, and cover with a lid.

- When the apples are soft, after about 5 minutes, strain and purée the apples.

- Mix in vanilla and cinnamon and set aside to cool.

- Separate the whites and yolks of the eggs and discard the yolks. Beat the egg whites to stiff peaks and fold in the apples.

- Spoon into a dessert bowl or other small bowl.

- Sprinkle walnuts on top.

- Serve chilled.

Makes one serving.

Exchanges/Choices: 1 fruit, 1/2 other carbohydrate, 1 lean protein, 1 fat
Per serving: Calories 179, Calories from Fat 46, Total Fat 5.1 g, Saturated Fat 0.5 g,
Monounsaturated Fat 0.7 g, Cholesterol 0 mg, Protein 8.7 g, Carbohydrates 24.9 g, Dietary
Fiber 4.2 g, Sugars 18.7 g, Sodium 111 mg, Potassium 289 mg, Phosphorus 51 mg

Shopping List:

1 apple
1 jar honey
1 package unsalted walnut pieces

Staples:

sugar substitute
vanilla extract
ground cinnamon
pasteurized eggs

Shop Smart

- Sugar substitute of your choice (I have used several different brands in creating the recipes)

Cinnamon Streusel Baked Apple

*The aroma of baking apples and cinnamon fill the
air when making this simple dessert.*

Helpful Hints

- Use an apple that keeps it shape when cooked such as Rome, Granny Smith, Cortland, or Braeburn.

> 1/2 cup sliced apple
> 1 teaspoon canola oil
> 1/2 tablespoon honey
> 1 tablespoon whole-wheat flour
> 1/8 teaspoon ground cinnamon
> 1/2 tablespoon unsalted walnuts pieces

- Preheat oven to 350°F.

- Cut apple in half, remove the core, and cut into 1/2-inch slices. Place the apple slices in a ramekin (about 3 inches in diameter and 1 1/2 inches deep) or an oven-proof dish (4 inches in diameter and 1 inch deep).

- Mix the oil and honey together in a small bowl until smooth. Add the flour, cinnamon, and walnuts. Mix well.

- Spoon the mixture in clumps over the apple slices.

- Bake 30 minutes or until the topping is golden and crisp.

- Serve warm.

Makes one serving.

Exchanges/Choices: 1 fruit, 1/2 other carbohydrate, 2 fat
Per serving: Calories 179, Calories from Fat 86, Total Fat 9.6 g, Saturated Fat 0.8 g,
Monounsaturated Fat 3.5 g, Cholesterol 0 mg, Protein 2.3 g, Carbohydrates 23.9 g,
Dietary Fiber 3.0 g, Sugars 15.4 g, Sodium 1 mg, Potassium 133 mg, Phosphorus 60 mg

Shopping List:

1 apple
1 small bag whole-wheat flour
1 small package unsalted walnuts pieces

Staples:

canola oil
honey
ground cinnamon

Fennel Apple Sauté

Savory and sweet flavors come together in this tasty recipe. Allen Susser, recipient of the James Beard award, gave me the idea for this quick, tasty recipe.

Helpful Hints

■ Rome, Granny Smith, Cortland, or Braeburn apples can be used instead of Red Delicious apple.

> 1/2 cup sliced Red Delicious apple
> 1 teaspoon olive oil
> 1/2 teaspoon fennel seeds
> 1/4 cup nonfat ricotta cheese
> 1/2 tablespoon honey

■ Cut apple in half, remove the core, and slice.

■ Heat olive oil in a skillet, add apple slices in one layer, then add the fennel seeds.

■ Sauté 2 to 3 minutes, turning slices over 1 to 2 times, or until the apples are soft but hold their shape.

■ Place the ricotta cheese in a dessert bowl, spoon apples and fennel seeds on top, and drizzle the honey over the apples.

Makes one serving.

Exchanges/Choices: 1 fruit, 1/2 other carbohydrate, 1/2 lean protein, 1 fat
Per serving: Calories 158, Calories from Fat 43, Total Fat 4.8 g, Saturated Fat 0.6 g,
Monounsaturated Fat 3.4 g, Cholesterol 0 mg, Protein 5.3 g, Carbohydrates 22.8 g, Dietary
Fiber 1.9 g, Sugars 17.1 g, Sodium 67 mg, Potassium 166 mg, Phosphorus 125 mg

Shopping List:

1 Red Delicious apple
1 small bottle fennel seeds
1 carton nonfat ricotta cheese

Staples:

olive oil
honey

Shop Smart

■ Nonfat ricotta cheese with 200 calories, 20.0 g protein, 20.0 g carbohydrates, 260 mg sodium per cup

Honey Cinnamon Apples

This apple dessert can be ready in 5 minutes with the help of a microwave oven.

Helpful Hints

- Rome, Granny Smith, Cortland, or Braeburn apples can be used instead of Red Delicious.
- Microwave ovens have different powers. Check the apple after 1 minute to see if it is soft.
- Watch the pecans carefully while they toast to prevent them from burning.

> 1 cup diced Red Delicious apple
> 1/2 teaspoon ground cinnamon
> 1/2 tablespoon honey
> 1 tablespoon dry-roasted, unsalted pecan pieces (1/4 ounce), toasted

- Cut apple in half, remove the core, and dice into 1-inch pieces. Place in a microwaveable bowl. Sprinkle cinnamon and honey over apple and toss well. Microwave on high 2 minutes.

- Spoon into a dessert dish and sprinkle pecans on top. Cool slightly before serving.

Makes one serving.

Exchanges/Choices: 1 fruit, 1/2 other carbohydrate, 1 fat
Per serving: Calories 148, Calories from Fat 47, Total Fat 5.2 g, Saturated Fat 0.5 g,
Monounsaturated Fat 3.0 g, Cholesterol 0 mg, Protein 1.0 g, Carbohydrates 27.9 g,
Dietary Fiber 4.3 g, Sugars 21.9 g, Sodium 2 mg, Potassium 174 mg, Phosphorus 35 mg

Shopping List:
1 Red Delicious apple
1 package dry-roasted, unsalted pecan
    pieces

Staples:
ground cinnamon
honey

Peanut Butter Apple "S'mores"

Peanut butter helps create a new flavor for popular s'mores in this recipe.

Helpful Hints

- The apples that work best here are ones that hold their shape such as Rome, Granny Smith, Cortland, and Braeburn.
- Whipped topping should be defrosted in the refrigerator for several hours before using.

> 1/4 cup sliced apple
> 1 tablespoon no-sugar-added peanut butter
> 1 tablespoon frozen, nonfat whipped topping (such as Cool Whip), defrosted
> 1/8 teaspoon ground cinnamon
> 1 graham cracker (2 1/2-inch square)

- Cut apple in half, remove the core, and slice. Place on a microwave-safe plate and cover with another plate or plastic wrap. Microwave on high 1 minute. Drain apples on paper towel.

- Mix peanut butter, whipped topping, and cinnamon together. Spread peanut butter mixture over graham cracker. Layer apple slices over peanut butter.

Makes one serving.

Exchanges/Choices: 1 fruit, 2 fat
Per serving: Calories 151, Calories from Fat 84, Total Fat 9.4 g, Saturated Fat 1.9 g, Monounsaturated Fat 4.0 g, Cholesterol 0 mg, Protein 4.6 g, Carbohydrates 14.5 g, Dietary Fiber 2.4 g, Sugars 7.9 g, Sodium 39 mg, Potassium 168 mg, Phosphorus 65 mg

Shopping List:

1 medium-sized apple (Rome, Granny Smith, Cortland, or Braeburn)
1 jar no-sugar-added peanut butter
1 container frozen, nonfat whipped topping (such as Cool Whip)
1 small box graham crackers

Staples:

ground cinnamon

Shop Smart

- Frozen, nonfat whipped topping (such as Cool Whip) with 7.5 calories, 1.5 g carbohydrates per tablespoon

Banana Frozen Yogurt Pops

Keep a few of these frozen pops in the freezer for a quick dessert. It's a good way to use up ripe bananas.

Helpful Hints

- Whole pasteurized eggs can be found in most supermarkets.
- If pops are left in the freezer for several days, let stand at room temperature a few minutes to soften.
- Instead of frozen pops, freeze the mixture in small bowls.
- To test if the egg whites form stiff peaks, lift beater with a little beaten egg white on it. The egg white should not move when shaken lightly.

> 2 egg whites, separated from whole pasteurized eggs
> Sugar substitute equivalent to 2 teaspoons sugar
> 1 cup sliced ripe banana
> 1 cup low-fat banana yogurt

- Separate the whites and yolks of the eggs, discard the yolks, and beat egg whites until stiff. Add sugar substitute and beat again to form stiff peaks.

- Combine banana and yogurt in food processor then fold into the egg whites.

- Divide between two cups (about 3 inches in diameter and 4 inches tall) and insert popsicle stick into the middle of each one.

- Freeze until solid, about 3 to 4 hours, or eat immediately as pudding or mousse. To serve, push pop out of cup by squeezing the bottom or cut the cup away.

Makes two servings.

Exchanges/Choices: 1 fruit, 1/2 reduced-fat milk, 1/2 other carbohydrate, 1 lean protein
Per serving: Calories 163, Calories from Fat 20, Total Fat 2.2 g, Saturated Fat 1.3 g, Monounsaturated Fat 0.6 g, Cholesterol 8 mg, Protein 10.9 g, Carbohydrates 26.4 g, Dietary Fiber 2.0 g, Sugars 18.4 g, Sodium 142 mg, Potassium 609 mg, Phosphorus 198 mg

Shopping List:

1 medium-sized banana
1 container low-fat banana yogurt
paper cups
popsicle sticks

Staples:

pasteurized eggs
sugar substitute

Shop Smart

- Low-fat yogurt with 154 calories, 3.8 g fat, 12.9 g protein, 17.3 g carbohydrates, 172 mg sodium per cup

Banana Pudding

This is a tasty variation of an all-American banana dessert that has the sweet banana flavor without all of the extra calories.

Helpful Hints

- Whipped topping should be defrosted in the refrigerator for several hours before using.
- Freeze remaining banana for another time.
- Sautéing the bananas brings out their sweet flavor.
- To keep the banana's shape, use a fork to turn them while they sauté.

    1 teaspoon canola oil
    1/3 cup sliced ripe banana, cut into 1/4-inch slices
        (about 1/2 medium-sized banana)
    1/2 cup frozen, nonfat whipped topping (such as Cool Whip), defrosted
    1 vanilla wafer

- Heat oil in a small nonstick skillet over medium heat.

- Add the banana slices and gently sauté 30 seconds. Using a fork, carefully turn the slices over and sauté 10 seconds or until the banana slices are soft.

- Place half the banana slices in a dessert bowl.

- Spoon half the whipped topping over the banana slices. Spoon the remaining banana slices on top. Spoon the remaining whipped topping over the banana slices.

- Crumble the wafer and sprinkle on top.

Makes one serving.

Exchanges/Choices: 1 fruit, 1/2 other carbohydrate, 1 1/2 fat
Per serving: Calories 161, Calories from Fat 67, Total Fat 7.4 g, Saturated Fat 1.6 g, Monounsaturated Fat 3.9 g, Cholesterol 8 mg, Protein 1.8 g, Carbohydrates 23.7 g, Dietary Fiber 1.4 g, Sugars 13.1 g, Sodium 43 mg, Potassium 217 mg, Phosphorus 39 mg

Shopping List:

1 medium-sized banana
1 container frozen, nonfat whipped
   topping (such as Cool Whip)
1 small box vanilla wafers

Staples:

canola oil

Shop Smart

■ Frozen, nonfat whipped topping (such as Cool Whip) with 7.5 calories, 1.5 g
  carbohydrates per tablespoon

Chocolate Banana Slices

*Chocolate drizzled over a sliced ripe banana makes
a quick, easy, and very delicious dessert.*

Helpful Hints

■ Freeze remaining banana for another time.

1/2 ripe banana, thinly sliced
1 tablespoon dark chocolate chips

■ Place banana slices on a small dessert plate.

■ Place chocolate chips in a microwave-safe bowl and microwave on high 30
seconds.

■ Drizzle chocolate over the bananas.

Makes one serving.

Exchanges/Choices: 1 fruit, 1/2 other carbohydrate, 1 fat
Per serving: Calories 133, Calories from Fat 41, Total Fat 4.5 g, Saturated Fat 2.9 g,
Monounsaturated Fat 1.0 g, Cholesterol 0 mg, Protein 1.3 g, Carbohydrates 25.6 g,
Dietary Fiber 2.9 g, Sugars 16.7 g, Sodium 6 mg, Potassium 349 mg, Phosphorus 54 mg

Shopping List:

1 medium-sized banana
1 package dark chocolate chips

Shop Smart

■ Dark chocolate chips with 70 calories, 3.0 g saturated fat, 9.0 g
carbohydrates per 15 g

Walnut-Crusted Banana

This scrumptious dessert is easy to prepare in minutes in a microwave oven.

Helpful Hints

- To chop the walnuts, add them to the food processor while it is running.
- Freeze remaining banana for another time.
- Whipped topping should be defrosted in the refrigerator for several hours before using.

> 1/2 medium-sized ripe banana
> 1 teaspoon brown sugar
> 1 tablespoon unsalted walnut pieces
> 1 tablespoon frozen, nonfat whipped topping (such as Cool Whip), defrosted

- Halve banana lengthwise and place one half on a microwave-safe dish and sprinkle with the brown sugar. Chop walnuts in a food processor and sprinkle over banana. Cover with plastic wrap and poke several holes in the wrap to vent.

- Microwave on medium power until brown sugar melts and banana is hot, about 20 seconds. Carefully remove the plastic wrap and top with the whipped topping.

- Serve immediately.

Makes one serving.

Exchanges/Choices: 1 fruit, 1/2 other carbohydrate, 1 fat
Per serving: Calories 129, Calories from Fat 45, Total Fat 5.0 g, Saturated Fat 0.5 g,
Monounsaturated Fat 0.7 g, Cholesterol 0 mg, Protein 1.8 g, Carbohydrates 21.6 g,
Dietary Fiber 2.2 g, Sugars 13.0 g, Sodium 4 mg, Potassium 270 mg, Phosphorus 42 mg

Shopping List:

1 medium-sized banana
1 small package unsalted walnut pieces
1 container frozen, nonfat whipped
  topping (such as Cool Whip)

Staples:

brown sugar

Shop Smart

- Frozen, nonfat whipped topping (such as Cool Whip) with 7.5 calories, 1.5 g carbohydrates per tablespoon

Blueberry Freeze

You will end your meal with a smile with this thick, frozen blueberry treat.

Helpful Hints

- Look for pasteurized, liquid egg whites in the egg section of the market.
- Sugar-free grape jam or sugar-free blackberry jam can be used.

1 cup frozen, unsweetened blueberries
1/2 cup pasteurized, liquid egg whites
1/2 teaspoon ground cinnamon
1 tablespoon sugar-free grape jam

- Place frozen blueberries, egg whites, cinnamon, and jam in the bowl of a food processor and process until combined. It will have a soft frozen texture.

- Pour into a glass and enjoy. It can be kept for a half hour in the freezer.

Makes one serving.

Exchanges/Choices: 1 1/2 fruit, 2 lean protein
Per serving: Calories 168, Calories from Fat 7, Total Fat 0.8 g, Saturated Fat 0 g, Monounsaturated Fat 0 g, Cholesterol 0 mg, Protein 14.4 g, Carbohydrates 30.9 g, Dietary Fiber 4.7 g, Sugars 20.9 g, Sodium 204 mg, Potassium 328 mg, Phosphorus 38 mg

Shopping List:

1 package frozen, unsweetened blueberries
pasteurized, liquid egg whites
1 jar sugar-free grape jam

Staples:

ground cinnamon

Shop Smart

- Sugar-free grape jam with 18 calories, 7.5 g carbohydrates per tablespoon
- Pasteurized, liquid egg whites with 7.5 calories, 0 g fat, 1.6 g protein, 24 mg sodium per tablespoon

Deep Dish Blueberry Cream

Fresh blueberries are topped with a blueberry sauce to give this creamy dessert a bright, blueberry finish.

Helpful Hints

- A small ramekin or a small dessert bowl can be used for this recipe.
- The fresh blueberries should be washed and dried on paper towels before use.

1/2 tablespoon cornstarch
Sugar substitute equivalent to 2 teaspoons sugar
1/2 cup water
1/2 cup blueberries, divided
1/2 cup low-fat vanilla yogurt

- Mix cornstarch and sugar substitute in a small bowl. Add water to a saucepan and stir in cornstarch mixture. Bring to a boil over high heat and allow to thicken.
- Add 1/4 cup blueberries and boil 3 minutes. Remove from heat.
- Place yogurt in a small ramekin or dessert bowl. Spoon the remaining 1/4 cup blueberries on top. Spoon blueberry sauce over berries.
- Refrigerate until needed.

Makes one serving.

Exchanges/Choices: 1 fruit, 1/2 reduced-fat milk
Per serving: Calories 138, Calories from Fat 19, Total Fat 2.2 g, Saturated Fat 1.3 g, Monounsaturated Fat 0.6 g, Cholesterol 8 mg, Protein 7.0 g, Carbohydrates 23.9 g, Dietary Fiber 1.9 g, Sugars 16.8 g, Sodium 87 mg, Potassium 344 mg, Phosphorus 186 mg

Shopping List:

1 container cornstarch
1 container blueberries
1 container low-fat vanilla yogurt

Staples:

sugar substitute

Shop Smart

- Low-fat yogurt with 154 calories, 3.8 g fat, 12.9 g protein, 17.3 g carbohydrates, 172 mg sodium per cup
- Sugar substitute of your choice (I have used several different brands in creating the recipes)

Cherry Almond Cheese Treat

Sweet cherries and toasted walnuts flavor this quick dessert. The natural juices from frozen, unsweetened dark cherries form a sauce for the dessert.

Helpful Hints

- Cherries can be defrosted in the microwave.
- Watch the almonds carefully while they toast to prevent them from burning.

1/2 cup frozen, unsweetened, pitted dark cherries
1 teaspoon vanilla extract
1/3 cup nonfat ricotta cheese
1 tablespoon slivered almonds

- Place cherries in a microwave-safe bowl and microwave on high 1 minute.

- Mix vanilla into the ricotta cheese, then place in a small dessert bowl. Spoon cherries over cheese.

- Toast almonds in a toaster oven or under the broiler. Sprinkle over the cherries and ricotta cheese.

Makes one serving.

Exchanges/Choices: 1 fruit, 1/2 other carbohydrate, 1 lean protein, 1 fat
Per serving: Calories 179, Calories from Fat 42, Total Fat 4.6 g, Saturated Fat 0.4 g, Monounsaturated Fat 2.9 g, Cholesterol 0 mg, Protein 9.4 g, Carbohydrates 21.5 g, Dietary Fiber 2.7 g, Sugars 13.4 g, Sodium 87 mg, Potassium 345 mg, Phosphorus 209 mg

Shopping List:

1 package frozen, unsweetened pitted dark cherries
1 container nonfat ricotta cheese
1 package slivered almonds

Staples:

vanilla extract

Shop Smart

- Nonfat ricotta cheese with 200 calories, 20.0 g protein, 20.0 g carbohydrates, 260 mg sodium per cup

Mascarpone-Filled Figs

The Italian cheese mascarpone is a creamy, white cheese that is the base of tiramisu. Here it is served with sweet, fresh figs for a refreshing dessert.

Helpful Hints

- Arrange the figs on a small dessert plate in a circle with the stems pointing in for an attractive dish.

    1/2 tablespoon mascarpone cheese (1/4 ounce)
    1 1/2 tablespoons nonfat ricotta cheese
    2 fresh figs

- Mix mascarpone and ricotta cheese together.

- Cut figs in half from stem to bottom. Place figs on a dessert plate, cut side up.

- Spoon mascarpone mixture in the center of each half.

Makes one serving.

Exchanges/Choices: 1 1/2 fruit, 1/2 lean protein, 1/2 fat
Per serving: Calories 123, Calories from Fat 32, Total Fat 3.6 g, Saturated Fat 1.8 g,
Monounsaturated Fat 0.1 g, Cholesterol 9 mg, Protein 3.1 g, Carbohydrates 21.1 g,
Dietary Fiber 2.8 g, Sugars 17.0 g, Sodium 28 mg, Potassium 58 mg, Phosphorus 9 mg

Shopping List:

1 small container mascarpone cheese
1 small container nonfat ricotta cheese
1 small package fresh figs

Shop Smart

- Nonfat ricotta cheese with 200 calories, 20.0 g protein, 20.0 g carbohydrates, 260 mg sodium per cup

Port-Poached Figs

Port wine gives a rich, sweet flavor to fresh figs.

Helpful Hints

- Five-spice powder can be found in the spice or Asian section of the supermarket. It can be sprinkled on vegetables, combined with other spices as a rub for meats and poultry, or added to a stir-fry.
- Whipped topping should be defrosted in the refrigerator for several hours before using.

> 2 small fresh ripe figs, quartered
> 1/4 cup port wine
> 1 teaspoon honey
> 1 teaspoon balsamic vinegar
> 1/4 teaspoon five-spice powder or 1 star anise
> 1 tablespoon frozen, nonfat whipped topping (such as Cool Whip), defrosted

- Cut figs into quarters.

- Combine port wine, honey, balsamic vinegar, and five-spice powder in a small saucepan. Place over medium-high heat and bring to a simmer.

- Add figs and simmer 5 minutes. Remove figs with a slotted spoon and place on a small dessert plate.

- Reduce remaining port sauce by half (takes about 30 seconds) and spoon over figs. Add whipped topping.

Makes one serving.

Exchanges/Choices: 1 fruit, 1 1/2 other carbohydrate
Per serving: Calories 189, Calories from Fat 3, Total Fat 0.3 g, Saturated Fat 0.1 g, Monounsaturated Fat 0.1 g, Cholesterol 0 mg, Protein 0.9 g, Carbohydrates 31.9 g, Dietary Fiber 2.3 g, Sugars 24.7 g, Sodium 10 mg, Potassium 261 mg, Phosphorus 24 mg

Shopping List:

1 package fresh figs
1 bottle port wine
1 bottle balsamic vinegar
1 bottle five-spice powder
1 container frozen, nonfat whipped topping (such as Cool Whip)

Staples:

honey

Shop Smart

■ Frozen, nonfat whipped topping (such as Cool Whip) with 7.5 calories, 1.5 g carbohydrates per tablespoon

Cinnamon Grapefruit

Here is a different way to serve grapefruit without adding extra calories.

Helpful Hints

- Using a serrated knife, peel the grapefruit over a bowl to catch the juices for the sauce.

> 1/2 grapefruit, sliced
> 1/4 teaspoon ground cinnamon
> Sugar substitute equivalent to 2 teaspoons sugar

- Preheat broiler. Line a baking tray with foil or use a small oven-to-table dish.

- Peel grapefruit over a bowl to catch the juice. You should have about 1 ounce of juice.

- Place the half grapefruit on a cutting board. Using a serrated knife cut the grapefruit into three 1/2-inch slices.

- Place slices in a single layer on the lined pan. Sprinkle with cinnamon.

- Broil 3 minutes.

- Mix sugar substitute into the grapefruit juice in the bowl and spoon over warm grapefruit.

Makes one serving.

Exchanges/Choices: 1 fruit
Per serving: Calories 44, Calories from Fat 1, Total Fat 0.1 g, Saturated Fat 0.0 g,
Monounsaturated Fat 0.0 g, Cholesterol 0 mg, Protein 0.8 g, Carbohydrates 11.1 g,
Dietary Fiber 1.6 g, Sugars 9.2 g, Sodium 0 mg, Potassium 173 mg, Phosphorus 10 mg

Shopping List:

1 grapefruit

Staples:

ground cinnamon
sugar substitute

Shop Smart

- Sugar substitute of your choice (I have used several different brands in creating the recipes)

Tipsy Grapefruit

Triple sec, an inexpensive orange liqueur, mixed with the grapefruit adds a hint of orange and a little extra zing. Triple sec can be bought in small splits at most liquor stores.

Helpful Hints

- Any type of orange liqueur such as Grand Marnier or çuracao can be used.
- Watch the pine nuts carefully while they toast to prevent them from burning.

> 1/2 grapefruit, cut into segments (about 1/2 cup)
> 1 tablespoon triple sec
> 1 tablespoon pine nuts

- Cut skin and pith away from grapefruit. Cut in half and separate the grapefruit segments from one half with a serrated knife.

- Place segments on a small dessert bowl and sprinkle triple sec on top.

- Toast pine nuts in a toaster oven or under the broiler and sprinkle on top.

Makes one serving.

Exchanges/Choices: 1 fruit, 1 fat
Per serving: Calories 113, Calories from Fat 33, Total Fat 3.7 g, Saturated Fat 0.6 g, Monounsaturated Fat 1.4 g, Cholesterol 0 mg, Protein 1.5 g, Carbohydrates 14.3 g, Dietary Fiber 1.9 g, Sugars 8.4 g, Sodium 4 mg, Potassium 207 mg, Phosphorus 11 mg

Shopping List:

1 grapefruit
1 small bottle triple sec or other orange
   liqueur
1 small package pine nuts

Kiwi Berry Cup

This fruit cup is pretty, tasty, and an easy company pleaser.

Helpful Hints

- Any type of berries can be used.
- Kiwi-flavored yogurt can be found in some supermarkets. Raspberry yogurt works well as a substitute, or choose a yogurt to match the berries you are using.

> 1 kiwi, peeled and cubed
> 1/2 cup fresh raspberries
> 2 tablespoons low-fat raspberry- or kiwi-flavored yogurt

- Mix kiwi cubes and raspberries together. Spoon into a dessert dish.
- Spoon yogurt onto the middle of the fruit.

Makes one serving.

Exchanges/Choices: 1 1/2 fruit
Per serving: Calories 93, Calories from Fat 11, Total Fat 1.2 g, Saturated Fat 0.3 g, Monounsaturated Fat 0.2 g, Cholesterol 2 mg, Protein 3.1 g, Carbohydrates 19.6 g, Dietary Fiber 6.1 g, Sugars 11.1 g, Sodium 24 mg, Potassium 380 mg, Phosphorus 85 mg

Shopping List:

1 ripe kiwi
1 package fresh raspberries
1 container low-fat raspberry- or
  kiwi-flavored yogurt

Shop Smart

- Low-fat yogurt with 154 calories, 3.8 g fat, 12.9 g protein, 17.3 g carbohydrates, 172 mg sodium per cup

Key Lime Chocolate Chip Cream

Dark chocolate complements the tart key lime juice in this tangy sweet dessert. It can be made a day ahead. Serve it in a martini glass or other attractive glass.

Helpful Hints

- Whipped topping should be defrosted in the refrigerator for several hours before using.
- Lime juice can be used if key lime juice is not available.

> 1/2 cup frozen, nonfat whipped topping (such as Cool Whip), defrosted
> 1 tablespoon bottled key lime juice
> Sugar substitute equivalent to 2 teaspoons sugar
> 1 tablespoon dark chocolate chips, coarsely chopped, divided

- Mix whipped topping, key lime juice, and sugar substitute together. Reserve 1 teaspoon chocolate chips and fold in the rest.

- Spoon mixture into a glass and sprinkle reserved chocolate chips on top.

Makes one serving.

Exchanges/Choices: 1 1/2 other carbohydrate, 1 fat
Per serving: Calories 134, Calories from Fat 38, Total Fat 4.3 g, Saturated Fat 2.8 g, Monounsaturated Fat 1.0 g, Cholesterol 0 mg, Protein 0.6 g, Carbohydrates 22.7 g, Dietary Fiber 1.0 g, Sugars 12.6 g, Sodium 25 mg, Potassium 130 mg, Phosphorus 63 mg

Shopping List:

1 container frozen, nonfat whipped topping (such as Cool Whip)
1 bottle key lime juice
1 package dark chocolate chips

Staples:

sugar substitute

Shop Smart

- Frozen, nonfat whipped topping (such as Cool Whip) with 7.5 calories, 1.5 g carbohydrates per tablespoon
- Dark chocolate chips with 70 calories, 3.0 g saturated fat, 9.0 g carbohydrates per 15 g
- Sugar substitute of your choice (I have used several different brands in creating the recipes)

Mango Fool

When mangoes are in season, this is a fast, tasty treat.

Helpful Hints
■ Ripe peaches can be used instead of mangoes.

1/2 cup ripe mango, cubed
1/2 cup low-fat mango or other tropical fruit yogurt
1 small mint sprig

■ Fold the mango cubes into the yogurt and spoon into an attractive martini glass or dessert bowl. Arrange a mint sprig on top.

■ Refrigerate until 15 minutes before needed. Let come to room temperature before serving.

Makes one serving.

Exchanges/Choices: 1 fruit, 1/2 reduced-fat milk
Per serving: calories 127, Calories from Fat 20, Total Fat 2.2 g, Saturated Fat 1.3 g, Monounsaturated Fat 0.6 g, Cholesterol 8 mg, Protein 7.1 g, Carbohydrates 21.0 g, Dietary Fiber 1.3 g, Sugars 19.9 g, Sodium 87 mg, Potassium 425 mg, Phosphorus 188 mg

Shopping List:
1 ripe mango
1 container low-fat mango or tropical fruit
  yogurt
1 small bunch mint

Shop Smart
■ Low-fat yogurt with 154 calories, 3.8 g fat, 12.9 g protein, 17.3 g carbohydrates, 172 mg sodium per cup

Melon with Ouzo

Sipping ouzo in a café is a typical way to end the day in Greece. Ouzo is distilled from grapes and flavored with anise seeds. When diluted with water, it becomes cloudy and white. Here it is spooned over melon cubes for a quick dessert.

Helpful Hints

- Pernod or other anise-flavored liqueur can be used instead of ouzo.
- Small bottles of liqueurs can be found in most liquor stores.
- Buy precut melon cubes in the produce department or at a salad bar.

    1 cup cantaloupe, cubed
    Sugar substitute equivalent to 2 teaspoons sugar
    1 tablespoon ouzo (1/2 ounce)
    Mint leaf for garnish (optional)

- Place cantaloupe in a dessert dish.

- Mix sugar substitute and ouzo together and pour over melon.

- Let stand for 15 minutes. Stir a few times before serving.

- Garnish with mint leaf (optional).

Makes one serving.

Exchanges/Choices: 1 1/2 fruit, 1/2 fat
Per serving: Calories 110, Calories from Fat 3, Total Fat 0.3 g, Saturated Fat 0.1 g,
Monounsaturated Fat 0.0 g, Cholesterol 0 mg, Protein 1.4 g, Carbohydrates 19.5 g,
Dietary Fiber 1.4 g, Sugars 18.9, Sodium 26 mg, Potassium 427 mg, Phosphorus 24 mg

Shopping List:

1 container cantaloupe cubes
1 small bottle ouzo
1 bunch mint (optional)

Staples:

sugar substitute

Shop Smart

- Sugar substitute of your choice (I have used several different brands in creating the recipes)

Orange Chiffon

*Fresh orange zest adds extra orange flavor to this light,
airy dessert. It's like biting into an orange cloud.*

Helpful Hints

- Whole pasteurized eggs can be found in most supermarkets.
- To zest an orange, scrape the skin with a zester or potato peeler.
- Zest the orange into the mixing bowl to capture the orange essence as you scrape the skin.
- To test if the egg whites form stiff peaks, lift beater with a little beaten egg white on it. The egg white should not move when shaken lightly.

1/4 cup water
1 teaspoon unflavored gelatin
1/4 cup nonfat orange-flavored yogurt
Sugar substitute equivalent to 2 teaspoons sugar
1 orange
2 teaspoons orange zest
1/4 cup orange juice, from zested orange
2 egg whites, separated from whole pasteurized eggs

- Pour the water into a small bowl, sprinkle the gelatin over the water, and set aside to dissolve.

- Mix yogurt and sugar substitute together in a mixing bowl. Zest orange over the mixing bowl. Beat in the orange juice. Set aside.

- Place bowl with gelatin in a saucepan and fill the pan with water to come 3/4 up the side of the bowl. Heat water to dissolve gelatin. When gelatin is clear, stir it into the orange mixture.

- Place in the refrigerator to set, about 15 to 20 minutes.

- Separate the white and yolks of the eggs and discard the yolks. Beat the egg whites to form stiff peaks.

- Remove orange mixture from the refrigerator and stir a spoonful of whipped egg whites into it to soften slightly. Then fold the orange mixture into the remaining egg whites.

- Return to the refrigerator for 1 hour to set.

Makes one serving.

Exchanges/Choices: 1/2 other carbohydrate, 1 1/2 lean protein
Per serving: Calories 98, Calories from Fat 4, Total Fat 0.4 g, Saturated Fat 0.1 g,
Monounsaturated Fat 0.1 g, Cholesterol 1 mg, Protein 11.8 g, Carbohydrates 12.1 g, Dietary
Fiber 0.1 g, Sugars 10.7 g, Sodium 149 mg, Potassium 333 mg, Phosphorus 83 mg

Shopping List:

1 packet unflavored gelatin
1 container nonfat orange-flavored
  yogurt
1 orange

Staples:

sugar substitute
pasteurized eggs

Shop Smart

- Nonfat yogurt with 97 calories, 0.3 g fat, 17 g carbohydrates, 133 mg sodium per cup

- Sugar substitute of your choice (I have used several different brands in creating the recipes)

Oranges in Cherry Coulis

Sweet black cherry sauce forms a colorful bed for sweet orange segments. This dish is pretty as a picture.

Helpful Hints

■ Any type of chopped nuts can be used.

1/2 cup orange segments
1/2 cup frozen, unsweetened dark cherries
1 tablespoon coarsely chopped, unsalted macadamia nuts

■ Peel orange and slice over a bowl to catch the juice.

■ Defrost cherries for 1 minute in a microwave oven. Purée in a food processor, adding juice from peeled oranges, or press cherries through a food mill.

■ Spoon cherry sauce (coulis) onto a small dessert dish. Arrange orange slices on top. Sprinkle chopped macadamia nuts over the oranges.

Makes one serving.

Exchanges/Choices: 2 fruit, 1 fat
Per serving: Calories 150, Calories from Fat 59, Total Fat 6.6 g, Saturated Fat 1.0 g, Monounsaturated Fat 5.0 g, Cholesterol 0 mg, Protein 2.1 g, Carbohydrates 24.1 g, Dietary Fiber 4.5 g, Sugars 18.7 g, Sodium 0 mg, Potassium 357 mg, Phosphorus 43 mg

Shopping List:

1 orange
1 package frozen, unsweetened dark
  cherries
1 small container unsalted macadamia
  nuts

Peach Crumble

This crumble is made by warming peaches and topping them with a crunchy crust. It takes only minutes to make.

Helpful Hints

- For best results, be sure your peach is ripe. The flesh will give slightly when pressed.

> 1 medium-sized ripe peach, stone removed and sliced (about 1 cup)
> 1 tablespoon flour
> 1 tablespoon rolled oats
> Sugar substitute equivalent of 2 teaspoons sugar
> 2 teaspoons canola oil

- Place peach slices in a ramekin (about 3 1/2 inches in diameter and 1 1/2 inches deep) or small microwaveable bowl. Microwave on high for 1 minute.

- Mix flour, oats, and sugar substitute together and blend in the oil.

- Spoon over fruit and place under broiler, about 6 inches from the heat, for 4 to 5 minutes or until topping is golden.

Makes one serving.

Exchanges/Choices: 1 fruit, 1/2 other carbohydrate, 2 fat
Per serving: Calories 192, Calories from Fat 88, Total Fat 9.8 g, Saturated Fat 0.8 g,
Monounsaturated Fat 5.9 g, Cholesterol 0 mg, Protein 2.9 g, Carbohydrates 25.0 g,
Dietary Fiber 3.0 g, Sugars 13.8 g, Sodium 0 mg, Potassium 320 mg, Phosphorus 60 mg

Shopping List:

1 medium-sized peach
1 container rolled oats

Staples:

flour
sugar substitute
canola oil

Shop Smart

- Sugar substitute of your choice (I have used several different brands in creating the recipes)

Peach in Kirsch

Kirsch, a clear brandy distilled from cherry juice and pits, is used mostly in cooking fruit desserts. Cooking kirsch can be found in many supermarkets. It has more of an almond taste and is not real kirsch but works well for this recipe.

Helpful Hints

■ Any type of liquor or brandy can be used.
■ Nectarines can be used instead of peaches.

1 medium-sized ripe peach, stone removed and sliced (about 1 cup)
Sugar substitute equivalent to 2 teaspoons sugar
1 tablespoon kirsch

■ Place peach slices in a dessert bowl and toss with sugar substitute. Drizzle kirsch on top.

Makes one serving.

Exchanges/Choices: 1 fruit, 1 fat
Per serving: Calories 102, Calories from Fat 3, Total Fat 0.4 g, Saturated Fat 0 g, Monounsaturated Fat 0.1 g, Cholesterol 0 mg, Protein 1.4 g, Carbohydrates 15.6 g, Dietary Fiber 2.3 g, Sugars 13.7 g, Sodium 0 mg, Potassium 293 mg, Phosphorus 31 mg

Shopping List:

1 medium-sized peach
1 small bottle kirsch

Staples:

sugar substitute

Shop Smart

■ Sugar substitute of your choice (I have used several different brands in creating the recipes)

Peach in White Wine

This refreshing combination is a drink and dessert all in one.
First you eat the peach, then you drink the wine.

Helpful Hints

- Peaches are peeled for this recipe, but if in a hurry, simply slice them and add the wine.

    1 medium-sized ripe peach
    4 ounces white wine, chilled (Sancerre or Riesling)

- Bring a small saucepan of water to a boil over high heat. Add the peach. Remove the peach after 5 seconds and dip immediately into cold water to stop the cooking.

- Peel the peach, cut in half, and remove the pits. Slice the peach, place in a glass, and add the chilled wine. Serve immediately with a spoon.

Makes one serving.

Exchanges/Choices: 1 fruit, 2 fat
Per serving: Calories 157, Calories from Fat 3, Total Fat 0.4 g, Saturated Fat 0 g,
Monounsaturated Fat 0.1 g, Cholesterol 0 mg, Protein 1.5 g, Carbohydrutes 17.8 g,
Dietary Fiber 2.3 g, Sugars 14.1 g, Sodium 6 mg, Potassium 377 mg, Phosphorus 52 mg

Shopping List:

1 medium-sized peach
1 bottle white wine (Sancerre or Riesling)

Peach Sorbet

This sorbet has a delicate peach flavor and creamy texture without using cream. The secret is to work quickly to keep the frozen texture of the peaches.

Helpful Hints

- Pasteurized whole eggs can be found in the egg section of the supermarket.
- To test if the egg whites form stiff peaks, lift beater with a little beaten egg white on it. The egg white should not move when shaken lightly.

1 egg white from whole pasteurized egg
1/2 cup frozen, unsweetened peaches
1/2 tablespoon honey
Several drops almond extract
1 tablespoon water
1 tablespoon sliced almonds

- Separate the white and yolk of the egg and discard the yolk. Beat the egg white to stiff peaks and set aside.

- Place frozen peaches, honey, almond extract, and water in a food processor and blend to a smooth sorbet. Remove from food processor and fold into whipped egg white.

- For a soft sorbet, place in chilled dessert bowl, sprinkle almonds on top, and serve immediately.

- For a firmer sorbet, place in a bowl and freeze for 1 hour. Remove from freezer and stir to break up ice crystals. Return to freezer for 30 minutes. Sprinkle almonds on top and serve.

Makes one serving.

Exchanges/Choices: 1 fruit, 1 lean protein, 1 fat
Per serving: Calories 132, Calories from Fat 42, Total Fat 4.7 g, Saturated Fat 0.4 g, Monounsaturated Fat 2.9 g, Cholesterol 0 mg, Protein 6.2 g, Carbohydrates 18.2 g, Dietary Fiber 2.3 g, Sugars 15.8 g, Sodium 56 mg, Potassium 272 mg, Phosphorus 64 mg

Shopping List:

1 package frozen, unsweetened peaches
1 bottle almond extract
1 small package sliced almonds

Staples:

pasteurized egg
honey

Baked Stuffed Pear

Juicy, fresh pears baked with almonds, brown sugar, and dried cranberries make an attractive dessert with very little fuss.

Helpful Hints

- I used a Bosc pear for this recipe because they hold their shape well when poached, but any type of pear can be used.
- A quick way to remove the pear core is to scoop it out with a teaspoon.

> 1 small ripe pear
> 2 tablespoons slivered almonds
> 1 tablespoon dried cranberries
> 1 teaspoon brown sugar
> 1/2 teaspoon almond extract

- Preheat oven to 400°F.

- Cut pear in half lengthwise. Remove core and scoop out a 2-inch hole in the center of each half with a spoon or small melon scoop. Shave off a thin slice from the round bottom of the pear to help it sit straight. Coarsely chop scooped out flesh and place in a bowl.

- Add almonds, cranberries, brown sugar, and almond extract to the chopped pears in the bowl. Toss well.

- Place pear halves in a shallow baking dish skin side down. Spoon almond mixture on the pears.

- Bake 15 to 20 minutes or until pears are soft.

Makes two servings.

Exchanges/Choices: 1 fruit, 1 fat
Per serving: Calories 105, Calories from Fat 41, Total Fat 4.6 g, Saturated Fat 0.4 g, Monounsaturated Fat 2.9 g, Cholesterol 0 mg, Protein 2.1 g, Carbohydrates 15.4 g, Dietary Fiber 3.0 g, Sugars 10.3 g, Sodium 1 mg, Potassium 132 mg, Phosphorus 50 mg

Shopping List:

1 small pear
1 small package slivered almonds
1 package dried cranberries
1 bottle almond extract

Staples:

brown sugar

Pears with Raspberry Coulis

Coulis is a thick sauce made from puréed fruits or vegetables. For this quick dessert, puréed sweetened raspberries form a base for juicy, ripe pear slices.

Helpful Hints

- The raspberry seeds are left in this sauce, which is puréed in a food processor. If you prefer the sauce without the seeds, strain the raspberries through a fine sieve.

> 1/2 cup frozen, unsweetened raspberries, defrosted
> Sugar substitute equivalent to 2 teaspoons
> 1 small ripe pear, sliced (3/4 cup)

- Place raspberries and sugar substitute in the bowl of a food processor and process until smooth. If you do not have a food processor, press berries through a sieve.

- Spoon sauce onto two dessert plates.

- Cut pears in half and remove core. Cut into slices and arrange on sauce.

Makes one serving.

Exchanges/Choices: 1 1/2 fruit
Per serving: Calories 96, Calories from Fat 5, Total Fat 0.6 g, Saturated Fat 0 g, Monounsaturated Fat 0.1 g, Cholesterol 0 mg, Protein 1.1 g, Carbohydrates 24.2 g, Dietary Fiber 7.2 g, Sugars 13.8 g, Sodium 1 mg, Potassium 215 mg, Phosphorus 31 mg

Shopping List:

1 package frozen, unsweetened raspberries
1 small pear

Staples:

sugar substitute

Shop Smart

- Sugar substitute of your choice (I have used several different brands in creating the recipes)

Lemon-Lime Pineapple Slices

Assemble this sweet dessert in a few minutes by using fresh pineapple slices, lemon or lime yogurt, and pecans. Fresh pineapple slices are available in the produce section of the supermarket.

Helpful Hints

- Any type of citrus-flavored low-fat yogurt can be used.

1 slice pineapple, 1/2-inch thick
1/3 cup low-fat lemon or lime Greek-style yogurt
1 tablespoon unsalted pecan pieces

- Place a slice of pineapple on a dessert plate, top it with yogurt, and sprinkle pecans on top.

Makes one serving.

Exchanges/Choices: 1 fruit, 1/2 other carbohydrate, 1 fat
Per serving: Calories 133, Calories from Fat 59, Total Fat 6.6 g, Saturated Fat 1.3 g, Monounsaturated Fat 3.0 g, Cholesterol 4 mg, Protein 8.5 g, Carbohydrates 11.2 g, Dietary Fiber 1.4 g, Sugars 8.8 g, Sodium 32 mg, Potassium 195 mg, Phosphorus 126 mg

Shopping List:

1 container fresh pineapple slices
1 container low-fat lemon or lime Greek-style yogurt
1 small package unsalted pecans pieces

Shop Smart

- Low-fat Greek yogurt with 130 calories, 3.5 g fat, 7.0 g carbohydrates, 70 mg sodium per 6 ounces

Pears in Red Wine

Ripe pear slices pick up the flavors of the cinnamon-spiced red wine in this tasty dessert.

Helpful Hints

■ Pear juice from the skins adds more flavor to the spiced wine. Be sure to capture the pear juice as you peel the pears.

    1 small ripe pear, sliced (3/4 cup)
    1/2 cup dry red wine
    1 teaspoon sugar
    Sugar substitute equivalent to 2 teaspoons sugar
    1 cinnamon stick

■ Peel the pear over a bowl, reserving the juice. Squeeze the skins to extract more juice and discard the skins.

■ Cut the pear in half, remove the core, and slice.

■ Mix the red wine, sugar, and sugar substitute in a small saucepan. Add pear juice from bowl, cinnamon stick, and the pear slices. Spread the pears in the liquid to make sure all of the slices are covered by the wine.

■ Place the saucepan over medium heat. Bring the wine to a simmer and cook gently 5 minutes.

■ Remove pears and arrange in a small dessert bowl.

■ Continue to simmer the wine to reduce by half, about 3 to 4 minutes.

■ Remove cinnamon stick and spoon sauce over the pears.

Makes one serving.

Exchanges/Choices: 1 1/2 fruit, 2 fat
Per serving: Calories 181, Calories from Fat 2, Total Fat 0.2 g, Saturated Fat 0 g,
Monounsaturated Fat 0.1 g, Cholesterol 0 mg, Protein 0.5 g, Carbohydrates 24.3 g,
Dietary Fiber 3.3 g, Sugars 16.0 g, Sodium 5 mg, Potassium 272 mg, Phosphorus 40 mg

Shopping List:

1 small pear
1 bottle dry red wine
1 package cinnamon sticks

Staples:

sugar
sugar substitute

Shop Smart

- Sugar substitute of your choice (I have used several different brands in creating the recipes)

Spiced Pears

Add a little extra spice to pears by poaching them
in cloves and lemon-flavored water.

Helpful Hints

- Keep the liquid on a low simmer to prevent the pear slices from breaking.
- Watch the walnuts carefully while they toast to prevent them from burning.

1 cup water
Sugar substitute equivalent to 2 teaspoons sugar
4 whole cloves
4 strips lemon peel from 1 lemon
1 small ripe pear, sliced (about 3/4 cup)
2 tablespoons unsalted walnut pieces
1 sprig fresh mint

- Place the water, sugar substitute, cloves, and lemon peel in a small saucepan.

- Peel the pear over the saucepan to catch the juice and add the peels to the saucepan. Core and slice the pear lengthwise. Add the slices to the saucepan. Bring to a simmer over low heat and gently poach 10 minutes.

- While the pears poach, toast the walnuts in a toaster oven or under a broiler.

- Remove the pear slices and arrange in a circle on a dessert plate. Place a sprig of mint in the center of the plate.

Makes one serving.

Exchanges/Choices: 1 1/2 fruit, 2 fat
Per serving: Calories 167, Calories from Fat 91, Total Fat 10.1 g, Saturated Fat 1.0 g,
Monounsaturated Fat 1.4 g, Cholesterol 0 mg, Protein 2.8 g, Carbohydrates 20.2 g,
Dietary Fiber 4.9 g, Sugars 11.4 g, Sodium 6 mg, Potassium 186 mg, Phosphorus 63 mg

Shopping List:

1 bottle whole cloves
1 lemon
1 small pear
1 small package unsalted walnut pieces
1 bunch fresh mint

Staples:

sugar substitute

Shop Smart

- Sugar substitute of your choice (I have used several different brands in creating the recipes)

Grilled Pineapple with Ginger and Basil Sauce

Fresh ginger and basil perfume this pretty dessert, which is an adaptation of a recipe by Latin American celebrity chef Alfredo Oropeza.

Helpful Hints

- Sliced fresh pineapple can be found in the produce section of most supermarkets.
- Pineapple can be placed under a broiler instead of on a grill.
- Whipped topping should be defrosted in the refrigerator for several hours before using.

1 teaspoon fresh ginger, grated
1/2 tablespoon fresh basil leaves, chopped
1 teaspoon brown sugar
1 slice fresh pineapple, about 1/2-inch thick
Canola oil cooking spray
1/8 teaspoon ground cinnamon
2 tablespoons frozen, nonfat whipped topping (such as Cool Whip), defrosted
Fresh basil leaves for garnish

- Combine ginger, basil, and brown sugar in a bowl. Add the pineapple slice and let sit 5 minutes, turn, and let sit 5 minutes to allow flavors to absorb.

- Remove pineapple from the bowl, reserve the ginger mixture, and spray both sides with canola oil spray.

- Heat a stove-top grill and add pineapple. Grill for 3 to 4 minutes or until it has grill marks and is slightly caramelized, about 3 minutes. Turn and grill until it has grill marks on the other side. Sprinkle with cinnamon.

- Remove to a small dessert plate. Mix whipped topping into the ginger mixture and spoon on top of pineapple. Add basil leaves as garnish.

Makes one serving.

Exchanges/Choices: 1 fruit, 1 fat
Per serving: Calories 95, Calories from Fat 38, Total Fat 4.2 g, Saturated Fat 1.3 g, Monounsaturated Fat 1.9 g, Cholesterol 0 mg, Protein 0.7 g, Carbohydrates 15.3 g, Dietary Fiber 1.0 g, Sugars 12.1 g, Sodium 12 mg, Potassium 88 mg, Phosphorus 12 mg

Shopping List:

1 small piece fresh ginger
1 small bunch basil
1 container fresh pineapple slices
1 bottle canola oil cooking spray
1 container frozen, nonfat whipped
   topping (such as Cool Whip)

Staples:

brown sugar
ground cinnamon

Shop Smart

■ Frozen, nonfat whipped topping (such as Cool Whip) with 7.5 calories, 1.5 g
   carbohydrates per tablespoon

Pineapple and Pine Nuts

In this simple dessert, toasted pine nuts add flavor and crunch to ripe pineapple.

Helpful Hints

- Buy fresh pineapple cubes in the produce section of the market.
- Watch the pine nuts carefully while they toast to prevent them from burning.

2 tablespoons pine nuts
1/2 cup fresh pineapple cubes

- Place pine nuts on a foil-lined tray under broiler or in toaster oven for 1 minute, until golden brown. Toss pineapple and pine nuts together.

Makes one serving.

Exchanges/Choices: 1 fruit, 1 fat
Per serving: Calories 102, Calories from Fat 66, Total Fat 7.3 g, Saturated Fat 1.1 g,
Monounsaturated Fat 2.7 g, Cholesterol 0 mg, Protein 1.7 g, Carbohydrates 9.5 g,
Dietary Fiber 2.0 g, Sugars 5.4 g, Sodium 9 mg, Potassium 134 mg, Phosphorus 9 mg

Shopping List:

1 container pine nuts
1 container fresh pineapple cubes

Raspberry Almond Whip

Puréed raspberry sauce gives a rich flavor to this whipped raspberry treat.

Helpful Hints

■ Look for sugar-free, ready-to-eat raspberry gelatin or make sugar-free gelatin from a package.

> 1/2 cup frozen, unsweetened raspberries, defrosted (or fresh raspberries)
> 2 teaspoons sugar
> 2 tablespoons nonfat ricotta cheese
> 1/2 teaspoon vanilla extract
> 1 tablespoon slivered almonds
> 3/4 cup (6 ounces) sugar-free, ready-to-eat raspberry gelatin

■ Add raspberries and sugar to a food processor and process until raspberries form a sauce. Add the ricotta cheese, vanilla, and almonds. Process to combine ingredients.

■ Whip gelatin with an electric mixer and add ricotta cheese mixture. Whip again.

■ Spoon into a dessert bowl. Refrigerate to set, about 20 minutes.

Makes one serving.

Exchanges/Choices: 1 fruit, 1/2 other carbohydrate, 1 lean protein, 1/2 fat
Per serving: Calories 167, Calories from Fat 44, Total Fat 4.9 g, Saturated Fat 0.4 g,
Monounsaturated Fat 2.9 g, Cholesterol 0 mg, Protein 6 g, Carbohydrates 24.7 g, Dietary
Fiber 5.1 g, Sugars 12.7 g, Sodium 78 mg, Potassium 201 mg, Phosphorus 185 mg

Shopping List:

1 package frozen, unsweetened
  raspberries or 1 container fresh
  raspberries
1 small container nonfat ricotta cheese
1 small package slivered almonds
1 package sugar-free, ready-to-eat
  raspberry gelatin

Staples:

sugar
vanilla extract

Shop Smart

■ Nonfat ricotta cheese with 200 calories, 20.0 g protein, 20.0 g carbohydrates, 260 mg sodium per cup

Plum Meringue

Meringue covers the plums like a golden cloud. This dessert will end your meal with a smile.

Helpful Hints

- Whole pasteurized eggs can be found in most supermarkets.
- Peaches or nectarines can be used instead of plums.
- Be sure to whip the egg whites to stiff peaks.
- To test if the egg whites form stiff peaks, lift beater with a little beaten egg white on it. The egg white should not move when shaken lightly.

> 2 ripe plums, pit removed and sliced (about 1 cup)
> 2 egg whites, separated from whole pasteurized eggs
> Sugar substitute equivalent to 2 teaspoons sugar

- Preheat oven to 350°F.

- Place plums in ramekin (about 4 inches in diameter and 2 inches deep) or small microwaveable bowl. Microwave on high 1 minute.

- Separate the white and yolks of the eggs and discard the yolks. Place the egg whites in the bowl of an electric mixer and beat to soft peaks. Add sugar substitute and whip to stiff peaks.

- Spoon egg white into ramekin, making sure the egg white completely covers the plum slices.

- Place ramekin in oven for 5 minutes or until meringue is golden. Serve immediately.

Makes one serving.

Exchanges/Choices: 1 fruit, 1 lean protein
Per serving: Calories 102, Calories from Fat 4, Total Fat 0.5 g, Saturated Fat 0 g, Monounsaturated Fat 0.2 g, Cholesterol 0 mg, Protein 8.2 g, Carbohydrates 17.3 g, Dietary Fiber 1.8 g, Sugars 15.2 g, Sodium 110 mg, Potassium 316 mg, Phosphorus 32 mg

Shopping List:

2 plums

Staples:

pasteurized eggs
sugar substitute

Shop Smart

■ Sugar substitute of your choice (I have used several different brands in creating the recipes)

Pumpkin Pudding

This pudding has a taste of autumn, with nutmeg, cinnamon, and pecans flavoring the pumpkin.

Helpful Hints

- Be sure to buy pure canned pumpkin rather than pumpkin with spices and other ingredients.
- Watch the pecans carefully while they toast to prevent them from burning.

2 tablespoons 100% pure canned pumpkin
1/8 teaspoon ground cinnamon
1/8 teaspoon ground nutmeg
Sugar substitute equivalent of 2 teaspoons sugar
1/3 cup low-fat vanilla yogurt
1 tablespoon unsalted pecan pieces

- Mix together pumpkin, cinnamon, nutmeg, and sugar substitute. Fold into yogurt.
- Toast pecan pieces in a toaster oven or under a broiler until golden, about 2 minutes.
- Spoon pumpkin mixture into a small dessert bowl and sprinkle pecans on top.

Makes one serving.

Exchanges/Choices: 1/2 reduced-fat milk, 1/2 carbohydrate, 1/2 fat
Per serving: Calories 116, Calories from Fat 58, Total Fat 6.5 g, Saturated Fat 1.4 g, Monounsaturated Fat 3.3 g, Cholesterol 5 mg, Protein 5.3 g, Carbohydrates 10.4 g, Dietary Fiber 1.8 g, Sugars 7.9 g, Sodium 59 mg, Potassium 285 mg, Phosphorus 149 mg

Shopping List:

1 can 100% pure pumpkin
1 container ground nutmeg
1 container low-fat vanilla yogurt
1 small package pecan pieces

Staples:

ground cinnamon
sugar substitute

Shop Smart

- Low-fat yogurt with 154 calories, 3.8 g fat, 12.9 g protein, 17.3 g carbohydrates, 172 mg sodium per cup

- Sugar substitute of your choice (I have used several different brands in creating the recipes)

Raspberry Parfait

*This dessert can be made in the morning to serve in the evening.
It is perfect for company and looks great in a parfait glass.*

Helpful Hints

- Any type of berry can be used.
- Any type of low-fat yogurt can be used.
- Watch the pecans carefully while they toast to prevent them from burning.

> 1/2 cup fresh raspberries
> Sugar substitute equivalent to 2 teaspoons sugar
> 1 tablespoon unsalted pecan pieces
> 1/2 cup low-fat raspberry yogurt

- Purée raspberries in food processor and blend in sugar substitute.

- Toast pecans in a toaster oven for 1 minute or until brown.

- Scoop half the yogurt into a bowl or parfait glass. Spoon in half the sauce and then the remaining yogurt. Add remaining sauce on top. Sprinkle with the pecans.

- Refrigerate until ready to serve.

Makes one serving.

*Exchanges/Choices: 1 fruit, 1/2 reduced-fat milk, 1/2 fat
Per serving: Calories 161, Calories from Fat 66, Total Fat 7.3 g, Saturated Fat 1.7 g,
Monounsaturated Fat 3.5 g, Cholesterol 8 mg, Protein 7.8 g, Carbohydrates 17.8 g, Dietary
Fiber 4.6 g, Sugars 12.4 g, Sodium 87 mg, Potassium 408 mg, Phosphorus 214 mg*

Shopping List:

1 container fresh raspberries
1 small package unsalted pecan pieces
1 container low-fat raspberry yogurt

Staples:

sugar substitute

Shop Smart

- Low-fat yogurt with 154 calories, 3.8 g fat, 12.9 g protein, 17.3 g carbohydrates, 172 mg sodium per cup

- Sugar substitute of your choice (I have used several different brands in creating the recipes)

Chocolate-Dipped Strawberries

Sweet strawberries are drizzled with a rich, dark chocolate sauce for this luscious dessert. The chocolate enhances the flavor of the juicy strawberries.

Helpful Hints

- Use a spoon to cream together the cocoa powder and oil to form a thick paste.

      4 large strawberries
      1 tablespoon unsweetened cocoa powder
      2 teaspoons canola oil
      Sugar substitute equivalent to 2 teaspoons sugar
      2 teaspoons sugar
      1/2 teaspoon vanilla extract

- Wash strawberries, leave stems on, and place on paper towel to thoroughly dry, patting gently with the towel.

- Add cocoa powder and oil to a bowl and cream together making a stiff paste. Add the sugar substitute, sugar, and vanilla. Mix well to form a thick sauce.

- Place the strawberries in a small dessert bowl and drizzle the chocolate over them or dip strawberries into the chocolate and enjoy.

Makes one serving.

Exchanges/Choices: 1 fruit, 2 fat
Per serving: Calories 159, Calories from Fat 89, Total Fat 9.9 g, Saturated Fat 1.1 g, Monounsaturated Fat 6.0 g, Cholesterol 0 mg, Protein 1.6 g, Carbohydrates 18.2 g, Dietary Fiber 3.4 g, Sugars 13.1 g, Sodium 1 mg, Potassium 197 mg, Phosphorus 56 mg

Shopping List:

1 container strawberries
1 container unsweetened cocoa powder

Staples:

canola oil
sugar substitute
sugar
vanilla extract

Shop Smart

- Sugar substitute of your choice (I have used several different brands in creating the recipes)

Strawberries and Grand Marnier Cream

Liqueur complements the flavor of fresh fruit. In this recipe, the Grand Marnier adds a sweet, orange flavor to this dessert.

Helpful Hints

- Any type of orange liqueur can be used, such as triple sec or çuracao.
- Whipped topping should be defrosted in the refrigerator for several hours before using.

> 1 cup strawberries, hulled and washed, divided
>   (about 8 medium-sized strawberries)
> Sugar substitute equivalent to 2 teaspoons sugar
> 1 tablespoon Grand Marnier
> 1/4 cup frozen, nonfat whipped topping (such as Cool Whip), defrosted

- Remove one strawberry and set aside. Slice remaining strawberries and place in a small dessert bowl.

- Chop reserved strawberry, place in a small bowl, and toss with the sugar substitute and Grand Marnier.

- Mix in the whipped topping and fold together. Spoon sauce over sliced strawberries.

Makes one serving.

Exchanges/Choices: 2 fruit
Per serving: Calories 120, Calories from Fat 4, Total Fat 0.4 g, Saturated Fat 0 g, Monounsaturated Fat 0.1 g, Cholesterol 0 mg, Protein 1.0 g, Carbohydrates 21.4 g, Dietary Fiber 3.2 g, Sugars 9.9 g, Sodium 10 mg, Potassium 240 mg, Phosphorus 44 mg

Shopping List: Staples:

1 container strawberries   sugar substitute
1 small bottle Grand Marnier
1 container frozen, nonfat whipped
   topping (such as Cool Whip)

Shop Smart

- Frozen, nonfat whipped topping (such as Cool Whip) with 7.5 calories, 1.5 g carbohydrates per tablespoon

- Sugar substitute of your choice (I have used several different brands in creating the recipes)

Creamy Balsamic Strawberries

A small amount of balsamic vinegar gives an
intriguing flavor to these strawberries.

Helpful Hints

- Use good quality balsamic vinegar.
- Whipped topping should be defrosted in the refrigerator for several hours before using.
- Mix honey and vinegar together until honey is completely blended with the vinegar.

1 cup sliced ripe strawberries (about 8 medium-sized strawberries)
1 teaspoon honey
1 teaspoon balsamic vinegar
2 tablespoons frozen, nonfat whipped topping (such as Cool Whip), defrosted

- Place strawberries in a dessert bowl. Mix honey and balsamic vinegar together and then blend in the whipped topping. Drizzle over strawberries.

Makes one serving.

Exchanges/Choices: 1 fruit, 1/2 other carbohydrate
Per serving: Calories 89, Calories from Fat 4, Total Fat 0.4 g, Saturated Fat 0.0 g,
Monounsaturated Fat 0.1 g, Cholesterol 0 mg, Protein 1.0 g, Carbohydrates 20.7 g,
Dietary Fiber 3.2 g, Sugars 14.6 g, Sodium 7 mg, Potassium 242 mg, Phosphorus 39 mg

Shopping List:

1 small container strawberries
1 container frozen, nonfat whipped topping (such as Cool Whip)

Staples:

honey
balsamic vinegar

Shop Smart

- Frozen, nonfat whipped topping (such as Cool Whip) with 7.5 calories, 1.5 g carbohydrates per tablespoon

Strawberry Frozen Yogurt Cup

Fresh strawberries top frozen yogurt for this easy dessert
that takes less than 5 minutes to make.

Helpful Hints

■ Place dessert bowl in the freezer to get cold while chopping the strawberries. This will keep the frozen yogurt from melting as soon as it touches the dish.

> 1/2 cup fresh strawberries
> 1/2 cup low-fat strawberry frozen yogurt

■ Wash strawberries, remove stem, and coarsely chop. Place yogurt in a dessert bowl and sprinkle strawberries on top.

Makes one serving.

Exchanges/Choices: 1 fruit, 1/2 lean protein
Per serving: Calories 74, Calories from Fat 5, Total Fat 0.6 g, Saturated Fat 0.3 g,
Monounsaturated Fat 0.1 g, Cholesterol 3 mg, Protein 3.1 g, Carbohydrates 14.1 g,
Dietary Fiber 1.6 g, Sugars 9.6 g, Sodium 55 mg, Potassium 245 mg, Phosphorus 90 mg

Shopping List:

1 small container fresh strawberries
1 carton low-fat strawberry frozen yogurt

Shop Smart

■ Low-fat strawberry frozen yogurt with 99 calories, 0.9 g saturated fat, 18.3 g carbohydrates per 1/2 cup

Fruit Tart

Fresh strawberries and blueberries top this individual tart. It can be made ahead and easily doubled or tripled to serve at a dinner party.

Helpful Hints

- Use a dessert dish or small pie dish that is about 4 inches in diameter and about 1 to 1 1/2 inches deep.
- For another presentation, place a 4-inch ring on a plate and press the graham cracker crumbs into the bottom. Spoon the yogurt mixture over the crumbs and place in the refrigerator to set. Once set, gently remove the ring, and top with strawberries and blueberries.

> 1/2 teaspoon unflavored gelatin
> 1 tablespoon water
> 1 tablespoon graham cracker crumbs
> 1 teaspoon canola oil
> 1/4 cup nonfat vanilla yogurt
> 1/4 cup sliced strawberries (2 medium-sized strawberries)
> 1/4 cup blueberries

- Mix gelatin and water together in a small glass or cup and set aside.

- Crush graham cracker and place crumbs in a small pie dish or dessert bowl measuring 4 to 5 inches in diameter and about 1 to 1 1/2 inches deep. Add the oil. Mix well until the graham crumbs are coated with the oil. Press the crumbs into the bottom of the dish. Refrigerate while preparing other ingredients.

- Place the glass with the gelatin into a saucepan. Fill the saucepan with water just to reach 3/4 up the side of pan. Heat water over medium heat to dissolve the gelatin, about 1 minute. Once the gelatin is clear, stir it into the yogurt.

- Remove the pie dish from the refrigerator and spread the yogurt over the bottom. Return to the refrigerator for 5 minutes. Wash the strawberries and blueberries. Set the fruit on paper towels to dry. Remove the stems of the strawberries and slice lengthwise.

- Remove the dish from the refrigerator and arrange the strawberry slices around the edge and place the blueberries in the center. Refrigerate 10 minutes before serving. The tart can be eaten immediately or refrigerated until needed. Remove from the refrigerator about 15 minutes before serving.

Makes one serving.

Exchanges/Choices: 1 fruit, 1/2 fat-free milk, 1 fat
Per serving: Calories 131, Calories from Fat 49, Total Fat 5.4 g, Saturated Fat 0.5 g,
Monounsaturated Fat 3.1 g, Cholesterol 1 mg, Protein 6.1 g, Carbohydrates 16.4 g, Dietary
Fiber 1.9 g, Sugars 11.3 g, Sodium 66 mg, Potassium 192 mg, Phosphorus 81 mg

Shopping List:

1 box unflavored gelatin
1 box graham crackers
1 container nonfat vanilla yogurt
1 small container strawberries
1 small container blueberries

Staples:

canola oil

Shop Smart

■ Nonfat yogurt with 97 calories, 0.3 g fat, 17 g carbohydrates, 133 mg sodium per cup

Grilled Fruit Kabobs

Grilling fruit brings out its sweet flavors and caramelizes the natural sugars.

Helpful Hints

- You can buy small containers of mixed cut fruit in many produce departments. Or, just use the same amount of one type of fruit for the kabobs.
- All fruit cubes are cut to about 2 inches.

1 cube honeydew melon
1 cube cantaloupe
2 red seedless grapes
1 cube watermelon
2 teaspoons canola oil

- Place honeydew cube, cantaloupe cube, grapes, and watermelon cube on small wooden skewer. Brush the fruit on all sides with the canola oil.

- Place on grill or stove top grill for 2 minutes, turn and grill 2 minutes, and turn again for 2 minutes, making sure all sides of the fruit touch the grill.

Makes one serving.

Exchanges/Choices: 1 fruit, 1 1/2 fat
Per serving: Calories 131, Calories from Fat 82, Total Fat 9.2 g, Saturated Fat 0.7 g, Monounsaturated Fat 5.7 g, Cholesterol 0 mg, Protein 0.7 g, Carbohydrates 13.0 g, Dietary Fiber 1.1 g, Sugars 11.1 g, Sodium 11 mg, Potassium 217 mg, Phosphorus 14 mg

Shopping List:

1 container of mixed fruit with honeydew melon, cantaloupe, grapes, and watermelon or other fruit
1 small package wooden skewers

Staples:

canola oil

Very Berry Crepes

Crepes stuffed with fresh berries make an enticing, simple dessert.
You can buy ready-made crepes in most supermarkets.

Helpful Hints

- Strawberries can be substituted for raspberries.
- If ready-made crepes are not available, spoon the berries over small slices of store-bought angel food cake.
- If using frozen, unsweetened fruit, defrost and drain any extra liquid.

> 1/4 cup fresh raspberries or frozen, unsweetened raspberries
> Sugar substitute equivalent to 2 teaspoons sugar
> 1/4 cup blueberries
> 1 7-inch ready-made crepe (about 1/2 ounce)

- Purée raspberries and sugar substitute in a food processor or push through a sieve, removing the pulp.
- Place blueberries in the center of the crepe. Spoon half the raspberry sauce over the blueberries.
- Roll up the crepe and drizzle the remaining sauce over the top.

Makes one serving.

Exchanges/Choices: 1 fruit
Per serving: Calories 71, Calories from Fat 7, Total Fat 0.8 g, Saturated Fat 0.5 g,
Monounsaturated Fat 0.4 g, Cholesterol 5 mg, Protein 1.7 g, Carbohydrates 14.9 g,
Dietary Fiber 2.9 g, Sugars 5.9 g, Sodium 51 mg, Potassium 100 mg, Phosphorus 36 mg

Shopping List:

1 container raspberries
1 container blueberries
1 package ready-made crepes

Staples:

sugar substitute

Shop Smart

- Sugar substitute of your choice (I have used several different brands in creating the recipes)

Mocha Magic

Mocha Cream Cake

The mixture of coffee and cocoa with an added touch of rum gives a rich flavor to this creamy sauce. It goes well over cake, ice cream, or fruit.

Helpful Hints

- A small amount of rum is needed. If you don't have it on hand, 1 teaspoon vanilla extract can be used.
- Angel food cake can be found in the bakery department of most supermarkets. Cut one slice and freeze the remainder for another time.

1/4 cup plus 1/2 tablespoon fat-free milk, divided
1/2 teaspoon instant coffee
1/2 teaspoon unsweetened cocoa powder
Sugar substitute equivalent to 2 teaspoons sugar
1 teaspoon rum
1 teaspoon cornstarch
1 thin slice angel food cake (about 1 ounce)

- Warm 1/4 cup milk in a small saucepan over medium heat. Add the coffee, cocoa powder, and sugar substitute. Lower heat to low and cook to dissolve the coffee and cocoa powder. Stir in the rum.

- Mix the cornstarch with remaining 1/2 tablespoon fat-free milk and add to coffee mixture. Stir well and cook 30 seconds or until sauce thickens. Sauce should be thick but still of pouring consistency.

- Place cake slice on a small dessert plate and spoon sauce on top.

Makes one serving.

Exchanges/Choices: 1 1/2 carbohydrate
Per serving: Calories 125, Calories from Fat 4, Total Fat 0.4 g, Saturated Fat 0.2 g, Monounsaturated Fat 0.1 g, Cholesterol 1 mg, Protein 4.2 g, Carbohydrates 23.8 g, Dietary Fiber 0.7 g, Sugars 4.3 g, Sodium 239 mg, Potassium 164 mg, Phosphorus 169 mg

Shopping List:

1 container unsweetened cocoa powder
1 small angel food cake

Staples:

fat-free milk
instant coffee
sugar substitute
rum
cornstarch

Shop Smart

- Sugar substitute of your choice (I have used several different brands in creating the recipes)

Mocha Fudge Cake

Rich dark chocolate and coffee give this fudge cake its flavor.

Helpful Hints

- Whole pasteurized eggs can be found in most supermarkets.
- Use a spoon to cream together the cocoa powder and oil to form a thick paste.
- To test if the egg whites form stiff peaks, lift beater with a little beaten egg white on it. The egg white should not move when shaken lightly.

> 2 tablespoons unsweetened cocoa powder
> 2 teaspoons canola oil
> 1/2 teaspoon instant coffee
> 1/2 cup hot water
> Sugar substitute equivalent of 2 teaspoons sugar
> 2 teaspoons brown sugar
> 2 egg whites separated from whole pasteurized eggs

- Preheat oven to 350ºF.

- Mix cocoa powder and oil together in a small bowl to form a uniform paste.

- Mix 1/2 teaspoon instant coffee into 1/2 cup hot water and measure 1/2 tablespoon of coffee for the cake.

- Add the 1/2 tablespoon coffee, sugar substitute, and brown sugar to the cocoa. Mix well. The mixture will be stiff.

- Separate the white and yolks of the eggs and discard the yolks. Beat the egg whites until stiff peaks form. Stir 1 spoonful of the egg whites into the chocolate mixture to lighten the mixture. Fold in the remaining whipped egg whites.

- Spoon into a soufflé dish (1 1/3 inches high and 4 inches in diameter) or a Pyrex bowl (3 inches high by 6 inches in diameter).

- Bake in the oven for 8 minutes and serve warm.

Makes one serving.

Exchanges/Choices: 1 carbohydrate, 1 lean protein, 2 fat
Per serving: Calories 176, Calories from Fat 95, Total Fat 10.6 g, Saturated Fat 1.5 g,
Monounsaturated Fat 6.2 g, Cholesterol 0 mg, Protein 9.4 g, Carbohydrates 16.7g, Dietary
Fiber 3.6 g, Sugars 10.4 g, Sodium 114 mg, Potassium 286 mg, Phosphorus 90 mg

Shopping List:

1 container unsweetened cocoa powder

Staples:

canola oil
instant coffee
sugar substitute
brown sugar
pasteurized eggs

Shop Smart

■ Sugar substitute of your choice (I have used several different brands in creating the recipes)

Mocha Granita

A granita is like a sorbet, but it doesn't contain egg whites or cream. It has a grainy texture and is very refreshing.

Helpful Hints

■ Whipped topping should be defrosted in the refrigerator for several hours before using.

■ Regular or decaffeinated coffee can be used.

> 1 cup coffee (or mix 1 teaspoon instant coffee into 1 cup hot water)
> 2 teaspoons unsweetened cocoa powder
> Sugar substitute equivalent to 4 teaspoons sugar
> 1 teaspoon vanilla extract
> 2 tablespoons frozen, nonfat whipped topping (such as Cool Whip),
>   defrosted, for garnish

■ Mix coffee, cocoa, sugar substitute, and vanilla together.

■ Pour into a metal bowl and place in the freezer for 2 hours. When it has started to freeze, remove and beat with a whisk. Place back in the freezer until it is nearly frozen.

■ Remove again and beat. Return to freezer for 30 to 40 minutes.

■ Remove and spoon whipped topping on top. Serve immediately.

Makes one serving.

Exchanges/Choices: 1 other carbohydrate, 1 lean protein, 2 fat
Per serving: Calories 52, Calories from Fat 15, Total Fat 1.7 g, Saturated Fat 1.4 g,
Monounsaturated Fat 0.2 g, Cholesterol 0 mg, Protein 1.2 g, Carbohydrates 7.4 g,
Dietary Fiber 1.2 g, Sugars 4.4 g, Sodium 7 mg, Potassium 106 mg, Phosphorus 36 mg

Shopping List:

1 container unsweetened cocoa powder
1 container frozen, nonfat whipped topping (such as Cool Whip)

Staples:

coffee
sugar substitute
vanilla extract

Shop Smart

- Frozen, nonfat whipped topping (such as Cool Whip) with 7.5 calories, 1.5 g carbohydrates per tablespoon
- Sugar substitute of your choice (I have used several different brands in creating the recipes)

Mochaccino Squares

These are chocolate and coffee gellées—
or little jelled squares—with a burst of flavor.

Helpful Hints

- A 4-inch by 4-inch container is best for setting the gelatin. I used a small plastic storage container. A 4-inch diameter bowl can be used.
- Look for a sugar-free, nonfat instant chocolate-flavored pudding mix. There are several brands.

1/2 tablespoon unflavored gelatin
2 tablespoons cold water
1/4 cup boiling water
Sugar substitute equivalent of 2 teaspoons sugar
2 tablespoons sugar-free, nonfat instant chocolate-flavored pudding powder
1/4 cup black coffee (or 1/4 teaspoon instant coffee dissolved in 1/4 cup hot water)
1 tablespoon half and half

- Add gelatin to cold water and let soak for 5 minutes. Pour boiling water into the cold water and gelatin mixture to dissolve the gelatin.

- Stir in the sugar substitute, chocolate pudding powder, coffee, and half-and-half.

- Pour into container and refrigerate for 2 hours to set.

- Remove from refrigerator and cut into 1-inch squares.

Makes one serving.

Exchanges/Choices: 1 other carbohydrate
Per serving: Calories 72, Calories from Fat 18, Total Fat 2.0 g, Saturated Fat 1.2 g,
Monounsaturated Fat 0.6 g, Cholesterol 6 mg, Protein 4.0 g, Carbohydrates 9.5 g, Dietary
Fiber 0.6 g, Sugars 1.5 g, Sodium 297 mg, Potassium 157 mg, Phosphorus 182 mg

Shopping List:

1 box unflavored gelatin
1 box sugar-free, nonfat instant
   chocolate-flavored pudding powder
1 carton half-and-half

Staples:

sugar substitute
coffee

Shop Smart

■ Sugar substitute of your choice (I have used several different brands in creating the recipes)

Chocolate Lovers

Chocolate Pudding

Creamy and smooth, with a deep dark chocolate flavor and not too sweet, this chocolate pudding can be served warm or cold and it takes only minutes to make.

Helpful Hints

- Fat-free milk can be substituted for soymilk.

> 2 tablespoons unsweetened cocoa powder
> 1/2 tablespoon cornstarch
> Sugar substitute equivalent to 4 teaspoons sugar
> 1/2 cup vanilla soymilk
> 1 teaspoon vanilla extract

- Combine cocoa powder, cornstarch, and sugar substitute in a small saucepan. Add just enough of the soymilk to make a smooth paste, about 2 ounces. Gradually stir in remaining soymilk, stirring until smooth.

- Cook over medium heat, stirring constantly, until mixture begins to thicken and bubbles appear, about 2 minutes.

- Remove from heat and stir in vanilla.

- Pour into a dessert bowl and refrigerate to set.

Makes one serving.

Exchanges/Choices: 1 1/2 other carbohydrate, 1/2 lean protein
Per serving: Calories 138, Calories from Fat 32, Total Fat 3.6 g, Saturated Fat 1.1 g, Monounsaturated Fat 1.0 g, Cholesterol 0 mg, Protein 6.1 g, Carbohydrates 23.1 g, Dietary Fiber 4.5 g, Sugars 6.8 g, Sodium 66 mg, Potassium 314 mg, Phosphorus 144 mg

Shopping List:

1 container unsweetened cocoa powder
1 small carton vanilla soymilk

Staples:

cornstarch
sugar substitute
vanilla extract

Shop Smart

- Vanilla soymilk with 131 calories, 4.3 g fat, 8 g protein, 15.3 g carbohydrates, 125 mg sodium per cup

- Sugar substitute of your choice (I have used several different brands in creating the recipes)

Chocolate Chip Meringue Cookies

These light cookies are filled with chocolate chips and melt in your mouth.

Helpful Hints

- Be sure to beat egg whites to stiff peaks and fold chocolate chips to distribute throughout the whipped whites.
- To test if the egg whites form stiff peaks, lift beater with a little beaten egg white on it. The egg white should not move when shaken lightly.
- This recipe makes sixteen cookies. A serving is four cookies.

> 2 egg whites separated from whole eggs
> 1/2 teaspoon cream of tartar
> Sugar substitute equivalent to 4 teaspoons sugar
> 1/2 teaspoon vanilla extract
> 1 1/2 ounces dark chocolate chips (about 1/4 cup)

- Preheat oven to 250°F.

- Line a baking sheet with parchment paper.

- Separate the white and yolks of the eggs and discard the yolks. Beat egg whites with cream of tartar to form soft peaks.

- Add the sugar substitute and vanilla and beat again to form stiff peaks. Fold in the chocolate chips.

- Spoon mixture onto parchment paper to make 16 cookies about 1 inch in diameter.

- Bake 30 minutes. Test to see that the cookies are dry and easily removed from the paper. Turn oven off and let cookies stay in the oven for 10 minutes.

- Remove from oven and allow to cool completely before storing in an airtight container at room temperature.

Makes four servings (four cookies per serving).

Exchanges/Choices: 1/2 other carbohydrate, 1/2 fat
Per serving: Calories 63, Calories from Fat 29, Total Fat 3.2 g, Saturated Fat 2.1 g,
Monounsaturated Fat 0.8 g, Cholesterol 0 mg, Protein 2.2 g, Carbohydrates 7.3 g, Dietary
Fiber 0.7 g, Sugars 6.3 g, Sodium 31 mg, Potassium 150 mg, Phosphorus 30 mg

Shopping List:

1 small bottle cream of tartar
1 package dark chocolate chips

Staples:

eggs
sugar substitute
vanilla extract

Shop Smart

- Dark chocolate chips with 70 calories, 3.0 g saturated fat, 9.0 g carbohydrates per 15 g
- Sugar substitute of your choice (I have used several different brands in creating the recipes)

Chocolate Mousse

This chocolate mousse is light as a feather and has a deep, dark chocolate flavor.

Helpful Hints

■ Be sure to stir chocolate until it is a smooth paste.

■ Whole pasteurized eggs can be found in the egg section of the market.

■ To test if the egg whites form stiff peaks, lift beater with a little beaten egg white on it. The egg white should not move when shaken lightly.

> 2 tablespoons unsweetened cocoa powder
> 1/2 tablespoon cornstarch
> Sugar substitute equivalent to 2 teaspoons sugar
> 1/2 tablespoon sugar
> 1/2 cup fat-free milk
> 1 teaspoon vanilla extract
> 2 egg whites, separated from whole pasteurized eggs

■ Combine cocoa powder, cornstarch, sugar substitute, and sugar in a small saucepan. Add just enough of the milk to make a smooth paste, about 2 ounces. Gradually stir in remaining milk, stirring until smooth.

■ Cook over medium heat, stirring constantly, until mixture begins to thicken, about 1 to 2 minutes. Remove from heat and stir in vanilla. Set aside to cool.

■ Separate the white and yolks of the eggs and discard the yolks. Beat egg whites to stiff peaks.

■ Mix one large spoonful of egg whites into the cooled chocolate to lighten the mixture. Fold the chocolate into the egg whites.

■ Spoon into a dessert dish and serve or refrigerate until needed.

Makes one serving.

Exchanges/Choices: 1/2 fat-free milk, 1 other carbohydrate, 1 lean protein
Per serving: Calories 155, Calories from Fat 15, Total Fat 1.7 g, Saturated Fat 0.9 g,
Monounsaturated Fat 0.5 g, Cholesterol 3 mg, Protein 13.5 g, Carbohydrates 24.2 g, Dietary
Fiber 3.7 g, Sugars 14.5 g, Sodium 164 mg, Potassium 469 mg, Phosphorus 214 mg

Shopping List: Staples:

1 container unsweetened cocoa powder

cornstarch
sugar substitute
sugar
fat-free milk
vanilla extract
pasteurized eggs

Shop Smart

■ Sugar substitute of your choice (I have used several different brands in creating the recipes)

Chocolate Walnut Balls

Increase the recipe to make a few of these frozen yogurt balls and store the extras in your freezer to use for a quick dessert at a later date.

Helpful Hints

- Place measuring cup, mixing bowl, and dessert bowl in the freezer to get very cold before using. This helps to keep the frozen yogurt from melting while making the dessert.
- Other flavors of low-fat frozen yogurt can be used.

> 2 tablespoons coarsely chopped unsalted walnuts, divided
> 1/2 cup low-fat chocolate frozen yogurt

- Place half the walnuts on a plate. Measure frozen yogurt into a cold bowl and quickly mix remaining walnuts into the yogurt.

- Shape the frozen yogurt into a ball with two soup spoons and roll the ball in the walnuts on the plate to coat the outside of the ball.

- Place in a small dessert bowl and freeze immediately. Freeze at least one hour before use. It can be kept frozen for several days.

Makes one serving.

Exchanges/Choices: 1/2 reduced-fat milk, 1 other carbohydrate, 1 1/2 fat
Per serving: Calories 195, Calories from Fat 93, Total Fat 10.3 g, Saturated Fat 1.4 g, Monounsaturated Fat 1.5 g, Cholesterol 4 mg, Protein 6.3 g, Carbohydrates 20.3 g, Dietary Fiber 2.8 g, Sugars 12.1 g, Sodium 76 mg, Potassium 380 mg, Phosphorus 171 mg

Shopping List:

1 small package unsalted walnut pieces
1 small container low-fat chocolate frozen
  yogurt

Shop Smart

- Low-fat chocolate frozen yogurt with 99 calories, 0.9 g saturated fat, 18.3 g carbohydrates per 1/2 cup

Custard, Creams, Cakes, and More

Honey Walnut Greek Yogurt

*Thick, creamy Greek yogurt, sprinkled with walnuts and drizzled
with honey, makes a sweet, creamy, and very tasty dessert.*

Helpful Hints

- Greek-style yogurt can be found in most supermarkets.

  1/2 cup low-fat vanilla Greek-style yogurt
  1 tablespoon unsalted walnut pieces
  1 tablespoon honey

- Spoon half the yogurt into a small cup and add 1/2 tablespoon walnuts.
  Spoon remaining yogurt over the walnuts and sprinkle remaining walnuts
  on top. Drizzle honey over the walnuts.

Makes one serving.

*Exchanges/Choices: 1/2 reduced-fat milk, 1 carbohydrate, 1/2 lean protein, 1 fat
Per serving: Calories 205, Calories from Fat 65, Total Fat 7.3 g, Saturated Fat 1.9 g,
Monounsaturated Fat 0.7 g, Cholesterol 7 mg, Protein 13.4 g, Carbohydrates 23.3 g, Dietary
Fiber 0.5 g, Sugars 22.5 g, Sodium 51 mg, Potassium 215 mg, Phosphorus 191 mg*

Shopping List: Staples:

1 container low-fat, vanilla Greek-style   honey
  yogurt
1 small package unsalted walnut pieces

Shop Smart

- Low-fat Greek vanilla yogurt with 130 calories, 3.5 g fat, 7.0 g carbohydrates,
  70 mg sodium per 6 ounces

Floating Island
(Oeufs à la Neige)

This fluffy cloud floats on a custard base. It takes a few minutes to make this classic French dish, but it is worth the time. It can be made several hours ahead.

Helpful Hints

- If you have difficulty spooning the poached egg white into peaks, simply spoon any stray bits onto the mounds. They will stay put.
- If the custard curdles a little, strain it into the dessert bowls for a smooth sauce.
- To test if the egg white forms a stiff peak, lift beater with a little beaten egg white on it. The egg white should not move when shaken lightly.

> 6 ounces fat-free milk
> Sugar substitute equivalent to 2 teaspoons sugar
> 1/2 teaspoon vanilla extract
> 1 egg
> 1/2 tablespoon sugar-free grape jam

- Add the milk to a medium-sized saucepan and warm over medium heat. Add the sugar substitute and vanilla extract. Stir to dissolve the sugar substitute.

- Separate the egg, placing the yolk in a bowl and whisking the egg white in another bowl to stiff peaks. Gently spoon the white on top of the milk. Heat the milk until almost boiling, about 1 minute.

- Remove the pan from the heat and with a large slotted spoon turn the white over. Return the pan to the heat and cook again for 1 minute. Remove the pan from the heat and place the white on a plate. Try to form a mound with a peaked top. The poached white will drain on the plate.

- Beat the egg yolk. Very slowly pour the milk used to poach the white into the yolk, stirring constantly. Pour the mixture back into the saucepan and place over low heat. Stir constantly until the liquid begins to thicken, about 3 to 4 minutes. The sauce will coat the back of a spoon.

- Remove from the heat and pour into a bowl. Continue to stir until the sauce cools. Pour the sauce into a dessert bowl.

- Carefully lift the white island off the plate and float it on the custard.

- Mix grape jam until it is smooth and drizzle it over the egg white.

Makes one serving.

Exchanges/Choices: 1 fat-free milk, 1 medium-fat protein
Per serving: Calories 153, Calories from Fat 44, Total Fat 4.9 g, Saturated Fat 1.7 g,
Monounsaturated Fat 1.9 g, Cholesterol 190 mg, Protein 12.5 g, Carbohydrates 14.4 g,
Dietary Fiber 0.2 g, Sugars 13.3 g, Sodium 148 mg, Potassium 364 mg, Phosphorus 277 mg

Shopping List:

1 jar sugar-free grape jam

Staples:

fat-free milk
sugar substitute
vanilla extract
egg

Shop Smart

- Sugar-free grape jam with 18 calories, 7.5 g carbohydrates per tablespoon
- Sugar substitute of your choice (I have used several different brands in creating the recipes)

Honey Pecan Custard

Toasted pecans add even more flavor to this honey-flavored creamy creation.

Helpful Hints

- Pour hot milk very slowly into the egg mixture to prevent it from curdling or breaking down.
- Watch the pecans carefully while they toast to prevent them from burning.

Vegetable oil spray
1/2 cup fat-free milk
Egg substitute equivalent to 1 egg
1/2 tablespoon honey
1/2 teaspoon vanilla extract
1/2 tablespoon unsalted pecan pieces, toasted

- Preheat oven to 350°F.

- Spray a ramekin or custard cup (4 inches in diameter and 2 inches deep) with vegetable oil spray.

- Pour milk into a small saucepan and heat over medium heat to just before boiling. Do not boil. Remove from heat.

- Add egg, honey, and vanilla extract to a bowl and whisk together. Very slowly add milk, whisking constantly. Pour mixture into ramekin and place in a roasting pan. Fill pan with warm water to reach halfway up the ramekin.

- Bake 40 minutes. When you insert a knife, it should come out clean. The center will not be firm, but it will firm as it cools.

- Toast pecans in a toaster oven or under a broiler. Sprinkle on top of the custard.

Makes one serving.

Exchanges/Choices: 1/2 fat-free milk, 1/2 other carbohydrate, 1 medium-fat protein
Per serving: Calories 153, Calories from Fat 49, Total Fat 5.4 g, Saturated Fat 0.5 g,
Monounsaturated Fat 3.3 g, Cholesterol 3 mg, Protein 9.0 g, Carbohydrates 17.1 g, Dietary
Fiber 0.3 g, Sugars 16.2 g, Sodium 145 mg, Potassium 310 mg, Phosphorus 166 mg

Shopping List:

1 carton egg substitute
1 small package unsalted pecan pieces

Staples:

vegetable oil spray
fat-free milk
honey
vanilla extract

Marsala Cream Pudding

Marsala (Italy's famous, fortified sweet wine) adds an intriguing flavor to this creamy raspberry pudding.

Helpful Hints

- Sweet sherry can be substituted for Marsala. Or, use rum extract found in the spice section of the supermarket as a substitute.
- Only a small amount of Marsala is used. It can also be used in small amounts to add flavor to dishes such as veal or chicken Marsala.

1/2 cup frozen, unsweetened raspberries, defrosted
Sugar substitute equivalent to 2 teaspoons sugar
1/2 cup low-fat vanilla yogurt
1/2 tablespoon Marsala wine

- Blend raspberries and sugar substitute in a food processor. Place yogurt in a bowl and stir in the Marsala wine and raspberries. Refrigerate or serve immediately.

Makes one serving.

Exchanges/Choices: 1 fruit, 1/2 reduced-fat milk
Per serving: Calories 124, Calories from Fat 21, Total Fat 2.3 g, Saturated Fat 1.2 g, Monounsaturated Fat 0.6 g, Cholesterol 8 mg, Protein 7.2 g, Carbohydrates 17.7 g, Dietary Fiber 4.0 g, Sugars 12.2 g, Sodium 87 mg, Potassium 386 mg, Phosphorus 195 mg

Shopping List:

1 package frozen, unsweetened raspberries
1 carton low-fat vanilla yogurt
1 bottle Marsala wine

Staples:

sugar substitute

Shop Smart

- Low-fat yogurt with 154 calories, 3.8 g fat, 12.9 g protein, 17.3 g carbohydrates, 172 mg sodium per cup
- Sugar substitute of your choice (I have used several different brands in creating the recipes)

Tapioca Pudding

*This sweet pudding is a favorite from my childhood
and a wonderful comfort food.*

Helpful Hints

- Tapioca comes from the starchy roots of the tropical cassava tree, which is also known as the manioc tree. Unlike regular tapioca, which contains large pearl-like beads, quick-cooking tapioca consists of small grains and is simple to make.

> 1 tablespoon quick-cooking tapioca
> Egg substitute equivalent to 1 egg
> 1/2 cup fat-free milk
> Sugar substitute equivalent to 2 teaspoons sugar
> 1 tablespoon sugar-free orange marmalade
> 1/4 teaspoon ground cinnamon

- Add tapioca, egg substitute, milk, and sugar substitute to a small saucepan. Let stand 5 minutes. Bring to a boil over medium-high heat, constantly stirring. Remove from heat and let stand 10 minutes.

- Stir in marmalade and spoon into a small dessert dish. Sprinkle with cinnamon.

Makes one serving.

*Exchanges/Choices: 1/2 fat-free milk, 1 other carbohydrate, 1 lean protein
Per serving: Calories 121, Calories from Fat 1, Total Fat 0.2 g, Saturated Fat 0.1 g,
Monounsaturated Fat 0 g, Cholesterol 3 mg, Protein 8.7 g, Carbohydrates 24.3 g, Dietary
Fiber 0.8 g, Sugars 13.6 g, Sodium 141 mg, Potassium 301 mg, Phosphorus 158 mg*

Shopping List:

1 package quick-cooking tapioca
1 carton egg substitute
1 jar sugar-free orange marmalade

Staples:

fat-free milk
sugar substitute
ground cinnamon

Shop Smart

- Sugar-free orange marmalade with 18 calories, 7.5 g carbohydrates per tablespoon
- Sugar substitute of your choice (I have used several different brands in creating the recipes)

Mini Cheesecake

This light cheesecake is topped with a sweet grape glaze.

Helpful Hints

- Sugar-free grape jam can be found in the jam and jelly section.
- Be sure to process the mixture until it is smooth.
- Any small ovenproof dish can be used. Follow the dimensions given.

> Vegetable oil spray
> 2 teaspoons reduced-fat sour cream
> 1/4 cup low-fat cottage cheese, no salt added
> 1 teaspoon brown sugar
> Sugar substitute equivalent to 2 teaspoons sugar
> 1/4 teaspoon vanilla extract
> Egg substitute equivalent to 1 egg
> 1 tablespoon sugar-free grape jam

- Preheat oven to 350°F.

- Spray a ramekin or custard cup (3 1/2 inches in diameter and 1 1/2 inch deep) with vegetable oil spray.

- Combine sour cream, cottage cheese, brown sugar, sugar substitute, vanilla extract, and egg substitute in a food processor. Process until smooth. Spoon batter into prepared ramekin.

- Place in a roasting pan and fill the pan with warm water to cover halfway up the side of the ramekin.

- Bake 35 to 40 minutes. A cake tester should come out clean. Remove from water bath and set on a wire rack to cool.

- Melt grape jam in a microwave oven for 10 seconds. Stir and pour over the cooled cheesecake.

Makes one serving.

Exchanges/Choices: 1 other carbohydrate, 1 1/2 lean protein
Per serving: Calories 145, Calories from Fat 38, Total Fat 4.2 g, Saturated Fat 2.6 g,
Monounsaturated Fat 1.2 g, Cholesterol 14 mg, Protein 12.5 g, Carbohydrates 16.7 g,
Dietary Fiber 0.4 g, Sugars 13.2 g, Sodium 124 mg, Potassium 137 mg, Phosphorus 200 mg

Shopping List:

1 small container reduced-fat sour cream
1 small container reduced-fat cottage
  with no salt added
1 container egg substitute
1 small jar sugar-free grape jam

Staples:

vegetable oil spray
brown sugar
sugar substitute
vanilla extract

Shop Smart

- Reduced-fat sour cream with 20 calories, 1.8 g fat, 0.4 g protein, 0.6 g carbohydrates, 13 mg sodium per tablespoon
- Low-fat cottage cheese with no salt added with 163 calories, 2.3 g fat, 28 g protein, 6.1 g carbohydrates, 29 mg sodium per cup
- Sugar-free grape jam with 18 calories, 7.5 g carbohydrates per tablespoon
- Sugar substitute of your choice (I have used several different brands in creating the recipes)

Natilla (Spanish Custard)

This is a perfect last-minute dessert. You don't have to go to the supermarket for the ingredients. They are all staples.

Helpful Hints

- The dessert can be made a day ahead. Cover and refrigerate. Bring to room temperature before serving.
- If the custard has small lumps, strain. This may occur if the temperature is too high before the cornstarch is added.

1 egg
1/2 cup fat-free milk plus 1 tablespoon
Sugar substitute equivalent to 2 teaspoons sugar
1 teaspoon cornstarch
1/2 teaspoon vanilla extract
1/4 teaspoon ground cinnamon

- Add egg to small saucepan and whisk to combine yolk and white. Add 1/2 cup fat-free milk and sugar substitute and whisk together. Place over low heat to warm, about 1 minute. Do not boil or the eggs will curdle.

- Mix cornstarch with remaining 1 tablespoon milk and add to mixture. Bring to a simmer and stir 1 to 2 minutes or until custard thickens. Remove from heat and add vanilla extract.

- Stir until the custard starts to cool. Pour into a dessert dish and sprinkle cinnamon on top.

Makes one serving.

Exchanges/Choices: 1/2 fat-free milk, 1/2 other carbohydrate, 1 medium-fat protein
Per serving: Calories 140, Calories from Fat 44, Total Fat 4.9 g, Saturated Fat 1.6 g,
Monounsaturated Fat 1.9 g, Cholesterol 189 mg, Protein 11.0 g, Carbohydrates 11.3 g,
Dietary Fiber 0.4 g, Sugars 8.3 g, Sodium 129 mg, Potassium 290 mg, Phosphorus 231 mg

Staples:

egg
fat-free milk
sugar substitute
cornstarch
vanilla extract
ground cinnamon

Shop Smart

■ Sugar substitute of your choice (I have used several different brands in creating the recipes)

Index

Cherry Almond Cheese Treat, 18
Chocolate Walnut Balls, 78
Cinnamon Streusel Baked Apple, 6
Honey Cinnamon Apples, 8
Honey Pecan Custard, 84–85
Lemon-Lime Pineapple Slices, 37
Oranges in Cherry Coulis, 30
Peach Sorbet, 34
Pineapple and Pine Nuts, 44
Pumpkin Pudding, 48–49
Raspberry Almond Whip, 45
Raspberry Parfait, 50
Walnut-Crusted Banana, 15

O

orange marmalade
    Tapioca Pudding, 87
oranges
    Orange Chiffon, 28–29
    Oranges in Cherry Coulis, 30
ouzo
    Melon with Ouzo, 27

P

parfait
    Raspberry Parfait, 50
peaches
    Peach Crumble, 31
    Peach in Kirsch, 32
    Peach in White Wine, 33
    Peach Sorbet, 34
peanut butter
    Peanut Butter Apple "S'mores," 9
pears
    Baked Stuffed Pear, 35
    Pears in Red Wine, 38–39
    Pears with Raspberry Coulis, 36
    Spiced Pears, 40–41
pecans
    Honey Cinnamon Apples, 8
    Honey Pecan Custard, 84–85

Lemon-Lime Pineapple Slices, 37
Pumpkin Pudding, 48–49
Raspberry Parfait, 50
pine nuts
    Pineapple and Pine Nuts, 44
    Tipsy Grapefruit, 23
pineapple
    Grilled Pineapple with Ginger and
        Basil Sauce, 42–43
    Lemon-Lime Pineapple Slices, 37
    Pineapple and Pine Nuts, 44
plums
    Plum Meringue, 46–47
Port-Poached Figs, 20–21
pudding
    Banana Pudding, 12–13
    Chocolate Pudding, 73
    Marsala Cream Pudding, 86
    Pumpkin Pudding, 48–49
    Tapioca Pudding, 87
pumpkin
    Pumpkin Pudding, 48–49

R

raspberries
    Pears with Raspberry Coulis, 36
    Raspberry Almond Whip, 45
    Raspberry Parfait, 50
    Very Berry Crepes, 59
red wine
    Pears in Red Wine, 38–39
ricotta cheese
    Cherry Almond Cheese Treat, 18
    Fennel Apple Sauté, 7
    Raspberry Almond Whip, 45

S

sorbets
    Peach Sorbet, 34
sour cream
    Mini Cheesecake, 88–89

soymilk
Chocolate Pudding, 73
Spiced Pears, 40–41
strawberries
Chocolate-Dipped Strawberries, 51
Creamy Balsamic Strawberries, 54
Strawberries and Grand Marnier Cream, 52–53
Strawberry Frozen Yogurt Cup, 55
streusel
Cinnamon Streusel Baked Apple, 6

T

tapioca
Tapioca Pudding, 87
Tipsy Grapefruit, 23

V

Very Berry Crepes, 59

W

Walnut-Crusted Banana, 15
walnuts
Apple Fluff, 4–5
Cheddar Apples with Walnuts, 3
Chocolate Walnut Balls, 78
Cinnamon Streusel Baked Apple, 6
Honey Walnut Greek Yogurt, 81
Walnut-Crusted Banana, 15

watermelon
Grilled Fruit Kabobs, 58
whipped topping
Banana Pudding, 12–13
Creamy Balsamic Strawberries, 54
Grilled Pineapple with Ginger and Basil Sauce, 42–43
Key Lime Chocolate Chip Cream, 25
Mocha Granita, 66–67
Peanut Butter Apple "S'mores," 9
Port-Poached Figs, 20–21
Strawberries and Grand Marnier Cream, 52–53
Walnut-Crusted Banana, 15
white wine
Peach in White Wine, 33
wine
Marsala Cream Pudding, 86
Peach in White Wine, 33
Pears in Red Wine, 38–39
Port-Poached Figs, 20–21

Y

yogurt. *See also* frozen yogurt
Deep Dish Blueberry Cream, 17
Fruit Tart, 56–57
Honey Walnut Greek Yogurt, 81
Kiwi Berry Cup, 24
Lemon-Lime Pineapple Slices, 37
Mango Fool, 26
Marsala Cream Pudding, 86
Orange Chiffon, 28–29
Pumpkin Pudding, 48–49
Raspberry Parfait, 50